Praise for *The Alchemy of Inner Work*

"*The Alchemy of Inner Work* shows the read
transparency and lucid presentation, ho'
body are necessary for the only healing
wholeness. The book vibrates with years
lifetimes of engaging the alchemical mystery of the creation of a
Self that has a body. I highly recommend it to both the general
reader and therapist alike."

—Nathan Schwartz-Salant, PhD, author of
The Mystery of Human Relationship

"True health is more than the elimination of symptoms; it is a recon-
nection of our bodies with our souls and spirits. This understanding
is urgently needed in our world. *The Alchemy of Inner Work* is a magnificent book, a gift for all who seek to transform suffering and disease
into well-being and wholeness, for themselves and for others. It is
the right book at the right time."

—Michael J. Gelb, author *of How to Think Like
Leonardo da Vinci* and *The Art of Connection*

"More pertinent today than ever, Lorie Dechar's *Alchemy of Inner Work*
skillfully weaves the timeless wisdom of the Tao into a life-changing
journey, touched with the intimacy of clinical experience. Combining myth, medicine, and magic, the book both comforted and
challenged me, as it worked its way into my cells to transform me as
only true alchemy can. What a masterpiece!"

—Randine Lewis, author of *The Infertility Cure* and
The Way of the Fertile Soul

"*The Alchemy of Inner Work* is a book for anyone who wants to awaken the inner healer to transform individual suffering. The book provides meditations and user-friendly tools to support readers in achieving a needed shift in consciousness—the key to alchemy—that can heal lives and help save our planet."

—Dr. Lorne Brown BSc, CPA, Dr.TCM, FABORM, CHt,
author of *The Acubalance Fertility Diet*

"It is a pleasure for me to endorse *The Alchemy of Inner Work*. My sincere hope is that everyone will read this treasure trove of essential inner knowledge. This book is a magnificent accomplishment."

—Caroline Myss, author of *Anatomy of the Spirit* and
The Power of Prayer

The
Alchemy
of
Inner Work

*A Guide for Turning Illness and Suffering
into True Health and Well-Being*

LORIE EVE DECHAR *with* BENJAMIN FOX

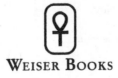

WEISER BOOKS

This edition first published in 2021 by Weiser Books, an imprint of

Red Wheel/Weiser, LLC
With offices at:
65 Parker Street, Suite 7
Newburyport, MA 01950
www.redwheelweiser.com

ISBN: 978-1-57863-686-0

Library of Congress Cataloging-in-Publication Data available upon request.

Cover design by Kathryn Sky-Peck
Interior by Debby Dutton
Typeset in Weiss and Proxima Nova

Printed in the United States of America
IBI

10 9 8 7 6 5 4 3 2 1

Dedication

To the unseen world that speaks to us
through a mystery.

And to Diana Chava and her generation,
who we do the healing for.

Disclaimer

In order to communicate the spirit of Alchemical Healing, I share stories about my own life as well as case studies drawn from my thirty-plus years of clinical practice. Except for accounts of my life or my life with Benjamin, the stories I present are "healing fictions," composite tapestries, woven from the threads of a variety of patients' experiences. My goal has been to offer a Body Felt Sense experience of the medicine while honoring the sanctity and privacy of the very personal work that happens in the treatment room. It is my hope that the people you encounter in these pages will be familiar to you as aspects of your own self, or friends you know or might have known, while remaining figments of the magical, mythical world of the imagination.

Alchemical Healing is not meant to be a replacement for diagnosis and treatment by a Western medical doctor or treatment by a licensed professional acupuncturist with years of advanced training, but it can support you in engaging with your own health care more effectively.

Contents

Part Three
Discovering Gold 191

Introduction

There is a language older by far and deeper than words. It is the language of bodies, of body on body, wind on snow, rain on trees, wave on stone. It is the language of dream, gesture, symbol, memory. We have forgotten this language. We do not even remember that it exists.

—Derrick Jensen, *A Language Older Than Words*

A young patient came to my office after having been hospitalized for an initial diagnosis of type 1 diabetes. At eight years old, he was doing his best to make sense of the experience, but he was having a hard time emotionally and his parents were worried.

"He just isn't himself," his mother told me when she called to arrange the appointment. "He isn't sleeping and he's lost interest in playing with friends. We think he's having trouble getting over what happened. We've heard you work with this kind of thing and we're hoping you can help."

Although insulin was now keeping my young patient's body functioning, another part of him still needed healing. This level of healing required more than acupuncture, more than herbs or medication. My patient needed a deep part of himself to be seen, heard, and related to. He wanted help transforming an overwhelmingly difficult experience into something meaningful, an event that he could potentially learn and grow from.

There were many hard feelings that he would clear through our conversations, but mostly he wanted me to know about the "bad stuff" had happened to him and how he thought things could have been handled better.

He told me about the sharp lancets they used "about a million times" to draw his blood, the things with prongs that went into his body, the special patient clothes he had to wear, and the pouches of fluid that hung over his bed. "But the very worst part of the whole thing," he told me, "the very worst thing of all"—and here he gave a hard, world-weary smile—"was the Ducky Band."

"The Ducky Band was a thing they put on your wrist, like the thing they put on merchandise in a store so you can't walk out with it. The band goes on with your name and what's wrong with you and it doesn't come off so you can't walk out even if you want to."

"I know they are trying to help you," he said, "but it feels terrible and they should know that. They put this band on your wrist and it's uncomfortable and it makes you know that you are sick. And then they stick this little yellow duck on it, because you are a kid, so they think this supposedly cute duck is going to make you happy, but it doesn't. A yellow duck doesn't make it all better."

"One experience like that," he said, "well, it takes about twenty of what I do with you to make it go away. Twenty, maybe even fifty, I don't know. But I think they need to understand because they forget how it feels inside."

Listening, I thought about another time—another era—when healers looked into their patients not with EKGs, blood tests, MRIs, and scalpels but with myths, stories, intuitions, touch, expanded sight, and dreams. So I decided to tell my young patient about another bird, a bird that isn't a cartoon character on a plastic band but a bird that flies through time and space and the mythic imagination. I told him the story of the marvelous Red Bird—the spirit animal of the Heart and Fire Element in ancient Taoist Healing.

"The Red Bird lives in your heart," I told him. "It is a little bird like a sparrow or wren. It is very friendly and likes to be near people. But when there is danger, this little bird grows big and fierce as a dragon and its wings spread out to touch the edges of the universe. When you need protection, you call his name and he flies out through a little door at the center of your chest. If you close your eyes and look

The Alchemy of Inner Work

inside, you might be able to feel that little door. You might be able to feel the door opening and the Red Bird coming out to greet you."

"Yes, I see him. He is spreading his wings wide open in front of me. He is flying out with big wide wings and sparkly black eyes, shiny and bright, protecting the whole front and back of me," he said.

"That Red Bird is always with you, no matter what happens," I said. "You can call on him whenever you get scared or need protection."

A few weeks later he came in with a jaunty smile and a battery-powered robot he was building himself. He told me he was feeling better. He had gone in for a check-up with the doctor and didn't get as upset as usual.

"It was still not great," he said. "They still made me go in that little room with no windows and tried to make me think it was okay because there were some games in there. There's just so much they don't understand. Like that stupid sign when you go in that says, 'Gate of Service.' What's that supposed to mean? Who do they think you are? A car filling up at a gas station or something? Vroom. Vroom. Fill me up!" Then he laughed uproariously. "Hey, I thought about the Red Bird. It helped. It's like that alchemy thing you were telling me about—turning lead into gold. Remember that from last time? So, the Red Bird helped me take something that felt bad and started to help me see how it could have some good in it."

"Like if I hadn't gotten sick, I probably never would have met you. And if I hadn't gotten sick, I wouldn't be learning about these special animals that give me my superpowers and other stuff that makes me feel better. Actually, I think those people at the doctor's office could really benefit from learning about this. You know, it could help them help people better, which I know is what they want to do. It could turn some things around. Hey, maybe you and me should start one of those, what do they call them, consultation companies, so we could teach people about this stuff."

The Red Bird allowed my patient to access something that was already in him but that he had lost touch with—his own resiliency and his capacity for courage, recovery, and growth. The Red Bird brought my patient back to himself in a new way. It allowed him to take a first step in changing his story and transforming his time in the hospital from one of confusion, upset, and fear to a difficult but meaningful experience that he could gradually integrate and understand. Eventually, it is possible that he will not only come to accept his chronic illness but will view it as the beginning of a new phase of his life, a doorway to a new sense of self and identity.

The story of the beginning of this young boy's recovery from a traumatic experience is only one of hundreds that my husband, Benjamin, and I can share about patients coming back to their lives—after illness, impasse, hardship, and loss—in new, more meaningful, effective, and joyous ways. Throughout our many years of work as healers and teachers, we have both come to believe that all change begins this way, by changing the way we see things. We both vividly recall when one of the participants of a workshop we were leading put it perfectly, exclaiming at the end of the four-day event, "It's my story. And I'm not sticking to it." He got it! Not sticking to our old stories and finding new ones is central to our work.

Benjamin and I practice and teach what we call modern-day alchemy. We emphasize *modern* because we are not hoping to return to some supposedly better long-lost past. Rather, we turn to the ancient myths, symbols, tools, and practices of alchemy to recover lost parts of ourselves. We seek to reawaken dormant ways of seeing, knowing, and imagining that will help us change the stories we tell. In this way, we hope not only to help ourselves and others but also to heal our world and create a future we want to be part of.

At this time in human history as we encounter crises of religion, race, politics, education, health care, economics, the environment, the prison industrial complex (PIC), and almost every other aspect of life on our planet, it becomes clear that our current worldview has reached an impasse. The promise of science and the rational mind as the solution to all our ills is no longer working. We long for resolutions to complex problems that have no simple fix. As the internet brings us into ever-increasing inter-connection, how will humans learn to get along and even cooperate with people who may think, look, or behave differently than they do? How can we justly apportion the

　　　　　　　　　The Alchemy of Inner Work

world's resources to give all beings a chance at life? What does it take to live a spiritually meaningful life? How can we care for ourselves without destroying our planet? What would it look like to restore the sacred to our considerations of health? And particularly important for modern Westerners, how can we assert our individuality and still feel part of a loving, caring, and interconnected community?

There is no doubt that we need to find new stories in every arena of modern life; however, the stories we share focus on health and healing. For us, the process begins not by fixing the medical insurance system, discovering better pharmaceuticals, or inventing more elaborate robotic technologies, but by changing the way we think, feel, and talk about ourselves and our world. The current conversations about health are stuck in endless feedback loops and the proposed solutions will not resolve the problems we face. Why? Because the questions we're asking miss the mark, arising from a too linear, quantitative, materialistic point of view that cannot begin to fathom the vast, multi-dimensional complexity of our lives and the challenges facing global change to health care.

The current cultural debate about healthcare is mired in a dualistic worldview that separates rather than connects, puts profit and the bottom line before empathy and relationship, and has no way to deal with the non-quantifiable dimensions of human experience. It leaves the innate wisdom and self-healing capacities of the body out of the conversation. Although modern Western medicine has achieved astonishing miracles in many areas, it was never meant to deal with every aspect of human suffering. As a good friend and devoted primary care physician said to me,

> "Western medicine is being asked to do too much. In the middle of everything else I have to do in the course of my day, I don't have time to teach people to listen to their bodies, to be self-aware, to figure out what really matters to them, so they have a reason to exercise, eat well, and generally take care of themselves. And yet that's the very thing that could interrupt the progression of most of the expensive, time-consuming, yet very preventable illnesses I treat."

My doctor friend was expressing frustration that she didn't have the time or the expertise to address the dreams, desires, and fundamental needs of her patients' souls or the wounds and losses that have led to their failure to know how to care for themselves. That isn't what she was trained to do, and it isn't in her job description. But it is what *we* do.

Through our work, we offer a redefinition of healing that brings the soul back into the conversation and links individual health to the vitality of the world soul—the surrounding community of human and nonhuman beings that make up our world. Alchemical Healing is not meant to be a replacement or even a complement to Western medicine, traditional psychotherapy, or the current symptomatic approach of modern Chinese medicine. Rather, it invites us to leap into a completely different conversation about health. It proposes a new set of values, attitudes, goals, and skills and offers a way to address the nonphysical forms of human distress, the psychic and spiritual imbalances, and dis-ease that are at the root of so much of modern suffering and illness. As my doctor friend says, "What you do doesn't complement Western medicine, it enhances it."

The increase in obesity, addiction, depression, anxiety, chronic pain, suicide, and innumerable other psychosomatic and mental health issues that are confounding our current health care system reinforces the importance of a new approach to psycho-emotional healing. We propose that there is a need for a healing process that honors the body as a source of wisdom, that is freely available, that engages people with their inner lives, that empowers us to understand our connection to the world differently. Such healing will enable us to respond to the challenges of our time in authentic, creative, and effective ways.

Whereas some people conclude that it is too late to turn things around, we take heart in the universal alchemical principal that without lead there can be no gold. In the midst of chaos, the new order can take form. As Benjamin and I remind each other on a daily basis, at times of death, the seeds of new life are already planted in the darkness and waiting for the right moment to push up into the light.

The Alchemy of Inner Work

Healing is a group activity. We need each other to see ourselves clearly, to reflect the changes we make, and to support us in keeping on course even when difficulties and challenges arise. The love, caring, and faith of our tribe is more potent medicine for the healing of our souls than any supplement or pharmaceutical. None of us can stay in a new story alone. It's too easy to slip back into belief systems that have defined us, language that has limited our experience, and the familiar patterns of thought and behavior. But if enough of us commit to standing for a new vision, it will become reality. That is how change happens. We must continually cultivate the new life that is emerging in order for it to flourish and grow. We need each other to do this. None of us can heal alone.

When I began writing this book, I assumed that I would write it by myself. After it was done, I imagined Benjamin would bring his relentless attention to detail to the editing and that would be that. But throughout the many years that this material as well as our work with Alchemical Healing has developed, it has become apparent that it takes a tribe to heal and transform the world. Benjamin, as well as our many patients and students, is as much a part of this book as I am. Although the case histories, stories, and much of the text is written in the first person by me, Lorie, Benjamin's editorial eye is behind every word. Every concept represents hours of shared conversation. And within every hope and dream that this book conveys are the years of effort that have gone into building our organization A New Possibility and the Alchemical Healing Mentorship community.

Benjamin and I have come to accept that this book is the child of our challenging and wonderful alchemical marriage. Right along with us, we include our alchemical community because we didn't give birth to this child alone and we won't be able to raise it without lots of help from our ever-growing extended family. Without mentioning specific names, we honor and thank our coauthors, all the courageous seekers who have worked with us in our clinical practices and the global community of acupuncturists, psychotherapists, body workers, nurses, doctors, and change-makers who have participated in our training programs and are actively engaged in visioning and manifesting a new medicine for the soul of our time.

We want to acknowledge at the outset the challenge we faced in weaving together these different voices, but we feel our efforts have been worthwhile. In our search to understand the new expression of human consciousness that we see erupting in the domains of ecology, spirituality, food sovereignty, the arts, gender, and sexuality and that we recognize as an intrinsic aspect of healing and survival at this time on the planet, we have come to believe that the future is multi-dimensional or as we like to call it, "integral." We are moving toward a consciousness that transcends our familiar ideas about time, space, and individual perspective, one that recognizes the uniqueness as well as the interrelatedness of all living beings.

In order to bring this emergent consciousness from implicit possibility into manifestation, we must bring fragmented parts together to form a new whole. We need to create new neural synapses, dismantle old structures, trust multiple truths, and see simultaneously from a variety of points of view. The leap to integrality requires the recovery of our natural human affinity for magic, myth, vision, and imagination without sacrificing our hard-earned mental capacity for critical thought and analysis of data. Our goals with this book are not only to share concepts and practices for improving the quality of your life but also to make our contribution to the global project of birthing this new consciousness.

This book is a hands-on workbook for anyone on a path of healing as well as a journey of discovery, a meditation on what it means to live a truly health-filled life. It is not meant to teach you to become an expert at a specific healing technique such as acupuncture, herbs, flower essence or essential oil therapy, counseling, or bodywork, although all these modalities will be included as useful tools. Instead, it is meant to help you understand and apply, in your own way, the principles, tools, and practices of alchemy and to discover how doing so can help you turn things around in your inner and outer world. Most of all, this book is an invitation to a new possibility and a reminder of an ancient memory—that we, like Alchemical Healers throughout history, have the capacity to imagine realities into being and to call the healing power of the soul into the world on a daily basis.

Part One

Modern-Day Alchemy

Chapter 1

Why Alchemy Now?

*... that darkness might be a medium of vision, and that descent may be
a movment towards revelation rather than deprivation.*

—Robert Macfarlane, *Underland*

An Alchemical Meeting

I discovered alchemy by accident. And yet, I now know that accidents can be the hand of destiny in disguise. At mid-life, I found myself in a trifecta of challenges, reeling from a year in the emotional combat zone of a difficult divorce and the daily breakdowns of an eight-year-old daughter whose family was coming apart at the seams. My former identity as an idealistic, reclusive poet and healer was crumbling in the face of the practicalities of material survival as a single mother and the greed, fear, and cruelty that had surfaced between me and my husband during the divorce process. I began having panic attacks, night sweats, and month-long bouts of insomnia as I perseverated over how I was going to mobilize my resources to find a new home, a new office, and a new life. In retrospect, I cherish the challenges—the financial uncertainty, emotional upheaval, and dissolution of identity—that I encountered at this time. I see now that these difficult experiences were not just meaningless suffering but rather the lead that was the basis of some of my life's most precious gold.

Around this time, I had a dream that I was walking around a dark square-shaped body of water. I had to make my way through the surrounding mud and grasses to get back to the place where I began so I could complete an important task that I could not yet name. After completing my passage along three sides of the pond, I came to the fourth side and saw that it was a shadowy marsh that appeared impossible to cross. I stood, hesitating at the edge of the fourth side, looking into the murky water. I wanted to go on but felt it was dangerous. After hesitating for a while, staring into the darkness, I decided to turn around, to walk the three sides back to the beginning rather than hazarding the uncertain waters alone. I realized that I needed help if I was going to make my way around the whole square. I would need new tools and information I did not yet have access to. I also knew that walking all the way around that square body of water was going to lead me not only to new ways of being with my patients but to a completely new way of being me.

Soon after having this dream, I met Nathan Schwartz-Salant, the person who would help me traverse the fourth side of the pond. Nathan had trained as a psychoanalyst at the C. G. Jung Institute, Zurich, and worked for decades as a psychoanalyst in New York City. Although he is recognized as a world-renowned Jungian analyst, I have come to realize that Nathan is fundamentally an alchemist.

There was nothing extraordinary about the conditions of my first meeting with Nathan. His office was located in a typical mid-rise Manhattan apartment building and looked like a standard therapist's office. There was a big green ficus tree in the corner, a long gray couch with pillows, and a chair upon which Nathan sat facing me across a few feet of beige carpet. What was unusual about the experience was that before walking through the door, I felt overcome by anxiety, shakiness, and uncertainty, but on leaving, my breathing had settled down, my heart had stopped racing, and I was no longer shaking. Nothing about the outer facts of my life had changed and yet I felt different.

What just happened?

What struck me first about Nathan was a quality of presence and weight. Sitting across from me on his leather recliner, he was with me in the way a stone or a tree is there, just being, with no need to know anything or to make anything happen. Yet, I felt I was being seen to my core, not just my surface self but all the way in to the shaking, terrified part deep inside of me. Within the safe confines of that room, I knew that I was with someone who could feel the confusion and grief that had been wracking my physical and emotional body and yet remain separate from it. This empathic sight was like a fine thread that wove my frayed edges and fragments back into a whole. Through that weaving, the empty, shaky parts of me began to fill in and settle down. I was landing back in my body after a long space flight. I felt my spine supported by the chair beneath me and the comforting pull of gravity for the first time in years.

After multiple acupuncture treatments, meditation retreats, massages, flower essences, herbal tinctures, counseling, and several rounds of different anti-depressant drugs in an attempt to work with my depression, anxiety, and upset emotional state, in one hour sitting in that room—with no physical touch, no needles, no herbs, no pharmaceutical drugs—my nervous system shifted gears. An inkling of hope penetrated my heart space. A tiny spark of faith rekindled.

The extremity of my emotional state combined with Nathan's insight and capacity for presence had allowed me to break through my impasse to a place outside the bounds of ordinary reality. In that altered state, I connected to a wiser and more resilient part of myself. At one point, I remember looking at Nathan's face and seeing another face appear. Although I was wide awake, it was as if I was also dreaming. Superimposed on his face was that of a big, patient black dog.

As soon as I caught a glimpse of the dog, I knew I had found my guide: a creature with a keen sense of smell and hearing, a creature with instincts to recognize the difference between danger and opportunity, and a creature cautious, wise, and courageous enough to find his way through the night forest. This creature was neither real nor unreal, not me or Nathan, but an imaginal being who appeared in the space between us as a wise woman's face emerges from the bark of a tree. As soon as I became aware of this animal's presence, my breathing shifted and I calmed down.

It was this co-created black dog guide—this earthy, savvy, loyal, hearty, nosy, magical creature—who would lead me back to the power of my own imagination and the wisdom of my body, who would give me the guts to speak my own strange truth, and who would bring me safely through the marsh on the fourth side of the square to a new sense of wholeness. It was only years later that I learned about the inexplicable synchronicity of Nathan's beloved black Rottweiler who passed away soon after we began working together. It was on that day, sitting on a gray couch with the dim Manhattan daylight filtering in between the partially closed Venetian blinds, that my alchemical journey began.

What Is Alchemy?

Although I didn't know it at the time, I later came to understand that the expanded state of awareness I experienced is the realm of alchemical consciousness. In this domain, the simplest of objects take on a dream-like significance. We recognize that the natural world is imbued with intelligence, that the boundary of the self extends far beyond the edges of our skin, and that not everything we experience can be understood or proven by the rational mind. It is in this domain of engaged presence, midway between the measurable realities of the material world and the immeasurable realm of spirit, that the soul—so long ignored by Western science and modern medicine—can heal and return to its rightful place at the center of our embodied lives.

Beginning that day and continuing until now with the writing of this book, I have been committed to understanding the subtle body shift that allowed me to begin to heal and find my way through the stress and trial of that time. My work is focused on finding concepts, skills, and practices that allow me to continue to heal myself and my patients, and to teach others to effectively work with this immaterial, immeasurable level of experience where so many of our modern Western disorders and symptoms arise.

I have studied various styles of acupuncture, herbs, flower essences, and essential oils as well as Zen Buddhism, Gestalt psychology, and a body-oriented awareness process called Focusing. I have read books on healing, consciousness, and the soul and studied the etymology of Chinese characters. I have been profoundly influenced by Carl Gustav Jung's archetypal psychology and post-Jungian work with psychic energy and relational fields.

I have come to understand that the unifying factor in all the theories and techniques I am drawn to is that they focus on a different level of experience than that championed by our current worldview, which prioritizes quantity over quality and splits the mind from the body. Although the systems I have been drawn to may not all explicitly use the terms *soul* or *psyche*, they all touch on this subtle level of being. They offer practices that allow us to consciously engage in what ancient adepts and healers called "inner work" or "soul work." I now recognize that this orientation was the central focus of an earlier knowledge tradition called "alchemy."

Alchemy is most simply described as the art and science of transformation. Alchemists sought to fundamentally change the nature of matter, specifically to upgrade the quality of something inert, corruptible, and opaque to something vital, enduring, and illuminated. By transformation, I don't mean the familiar change when we take a pharmaceutical to get rid of one symptom only to leave us with a host of annoying new side effects. Nor am I referring to change that moves along a one-way path toward degradation like the oxidation of metal, the rotting of vegetation, or other aging processes. By alchemical transformation, I'm not referring to only outer physical processes such as the combining of flour, yeast, and water into bread.

Alchemical transformation refers to processes that initiate and sustain growth, reverse entropy, and result in an upgrade on both outer and inner levels of experience. Alchemists sought to understand how structures, organisms, and systems could move toward more elegant, effective, and durable states rather than toward dissolution and degradation over time. Although the sole aim of alchemy is often said to be changing base lead into gold, its actual goal is to evolve a substance—whether metal, plant, or person—in order to extract or express its inherent divine nature. In other words, alchemists looked at how a substance or being moves closer to the fullest, most potent expression of its true nature.

To understand the wisdom and contributions of alchemy, it is not enough to say that it was a precursor to modern science. Although alchemy's influence on the development of modern Western science cannot be denied, the two systems have their own values, agendas, questions, and attitudes. In the words of biochemist and philosopher Mae-Wan Ho, modern Western science "[i]s dominated by an analytical tradition that progressively separates and fragments that which for many of us appears to be the seamless perfection that once was reality." Alchemy, on the other hand, throughout its many centuries of existence in India, Europe, China, and the Arab world, was dominated by a tradition of synthesis and integration. Nathan Schwartz-Salant writes in *The Mystery of Human Relationship,*

> Alchemy was based upon a belief in the fundamental unity of all processes in nature. All of nature—stone, metals, wood, and minerals along with the human mind and body—was formed out of a single substance. This essence, the lapis, was the basis out of which everything grew, and if one could gain some of it, even a minute drop, then considerable healing and transformation could be accomplished.

Alchemists asked the same questions that philosophers throughout time asked when confronted with the riddle of embodied life. Why do we suffer illness, loss, and death? Is there an afterlife? Do human beings have souls? What does nature consist of? Are human beings up to something in the cosmos? What is the meaning of a human life? And most importantly, is there a divine principle or essence that flows through all of life? If there is, how do we find it?

In keeping with the transformational intent and inquiring attitude of all alchemical traditions, Alchemical Healing, the alchemy described in this book, works to transform the suffering of our spiritual, emotional, and physical symptoms into meaningful messages that hold the potential to illuminate the divine purpose of life. The pressing question then, which I hear time and time again in my treatment room, is, "Am I living the life I was born to live?"

Historical Origins

Alchemical ideas and practices appear in the mystical traditions and perennial philosophies of a wide variety of cultures between 1000 BCE and 1800 CE. Although many alchemical texts have been lost or destroyed, enough remain to puzzle, entice, and inspire us. Bringing modern-day insight to bear on the still existing texts, we can begin to piece together a coherent view of alchemical consciousness.

Alchemy was the way that human beings in many cultures organized their observations of reality until modern science and dualism overshadowed alchemical awareness. The first stirrings of alchemy arose as shamanism declined during the Bronze Age. In both the East and the West, the initial movement from the nature-centered unity consciousness of tribal shamanism to the more objective laboratory experimentation of alchemy emerged around 2000 BCE with the development of smelting technologies and embalming techniques.

From the first millennium through the Renaissance, alchemy evolved steadily in Egypt, India, China, and Europe as human beings continued to explore their inner and outer worlds. As cultures developed the capacity to work with metals, document their histories, create calendars to predict the movement of the stars, and form vessels that could withstand high heat, a new perception of space and time emerged that included the awareness of past and future, above and below, within and without. People began to relate to the material world differently, to be curious about its properties, and to perform actions that significantly altered their environment. As alchemists explored the outer realm of matter through laboratory technologies, they also became increasingly interested in the possibilities inherent in their own being—the inner laboratory of the soul—and began to create elaborate practices to upgrade the value, durability, and luminosity of their own lives.

Chinese alchemy is entwined with the symbols and myths of Taoism, which along with Buddhism and Confucianism, is one of the three main spiritual traditions of China. European alchemy is heavily influenced by the Judeo-Christian mystical traditions; thus, its outer expression at first seems quite different from the Chinese. Yet, as I delved deeper into Taoist, European, and other alchemical systems,

I discovered overlapping insights, related symbols, and amazingly synchronous practices. Alchemical principles are at the root of Taoist, Kabbalistic, Christian mystical, and Buddhist meditation practices and also form the basis of traditional Chinese medicine and the modern depth psychology developed by C. G. Jung. I now believe that the alchemical worldview emerges from a universal stratum of human consciousness that is innate and crucial to our wholeness, though less in the foreground today than it was for human beings a thousand years ago.

Alchemy Today

I wake up early one tender green morning in late Spring, prepare myself a cup of tea, and open up the news feed on my computer. A headline from the *Washington Post* screeches out in bold letters across cyber space: "Suicide Rates Rise Sharply Across the Country, New Report Shows." I click on the link compulsively, remembering my thirty-year-old nephew who shot himself ten years ago, my beloved cousin's twenty-one-year-old daughter who bought a handgun and did the same, a friend's brother who died of a heroin overdose last month, another who went out on fentanyl, and thinking of the thousands and thousands of other radiant stars extinguished before they even glimpsed their own light. I forget about my tea and read further.

In a June 2018 *Washington Post* report, the Center for Disease Control and Prevention states that suicides have increased in all but one state between 1999 and 2016 across age, gender, race, and ethnicity. I click further and a cursory search of the internet reveals similar statistics about the dramatic rise in opioid addiction, vaping, obesity, pathological depression, and post-traumatic stress as well as the resulting associated health risks that are putting an impossible strain on our health care system. Yet, in a *New York Times* opinion piece that appeared in January 2018, Nicholas Kristof reports that "[t]he overall state of humanity is better now than at any time in history." In fact, Kristof asserts, 2017 was the best year ever for human health.

What is going on here?

In the modern world, most assessments of health care systems focus almost entirely on quantitative research and "evidence-based treatments" that rely on numbers and financial outcome to determine efficacy. Author and speaker Charles Eisenstein counters this perspective in an essay entitled "Our New, Happy Life? The Ideology of Development," written in response to Kristof's editorial. Eisenstein writes,

> Life expectancy . . . continues to rise globally . . . [however] these metrics obscure disturbing trends. A host of new diseases such as autoimmunity, allergies, Lyme, and autism, compounded with unprecedented levels of addiction, depression, and obesity, contribute to declining physical vitality throughout the developed world, and increasingly in developing countries too. Vast social resources—one-fifth of GDP in the US—go toward sick care; society as a whole is unwell.

If we want to create a world of truly healthy humans, I think we must begin by asking the question, "What is making us so sick?" What is sapping our young people's hopes and dreams and our elder's serenity and wisdom? What is draining resiliency, curiosity, innovation, joy, gratitude, and reverence from people's lives? The answers to these questions are, of course, complex. Yet, I believe at the root lies a loss of connection to soul. Current studies on the effectiveness of health care focus on quantity—how long can we keep people alive, at whatever cost—rather than on the quality of life. Death is viewed as the enemy to be beaten—our life victimized by the betrayal of our body—rather than our greatest teacher and an ever-present reminder of the preciousness of each moment in life.

This way of thinking—one that separates and insists on asserting dominance over nature and the natural unfolding of life and death—is felt in every aspect of our society. It has come to a head, however, in the field of medicine. As the unsustainability of our current health care system becomes increasingly obvious, medicine has become a "hot spot" where the need for a new, expanded way of organizing reality is strikingly apparent. As hospitals, medical centers, and insurance companies struggle to maintain their capacity to respond to the realities of human suffering, these institutions are suffocating beneath mountains of bureaucracy, malpractice suits, and rising costs. Meanwhile, larger portions of the population are spending vast sums of out-of-pocket money on "alternative" methods of healing that have not yet been accepted by these established institutions. A patient of mine complained that she is consistently referred to various specialists who only relate to a single part of her. She is not alone. People in my care are often relieved when they discover a relationship that considers the whole of who they are—physically, emotionally, and spiritually.

As a spiritual science, alchemy has always invited us deeply into the world. It involves our full engagement with organic life on Earth—with our bodies and with the communities of other beings—while consciously employing practices, tools, and substances that activate inner psychic experience. Alchemy includes the healing power of the imagination, it insists on the dynamic field created through relationship, and it invites spirit into the experience of being human. It is through such conscious and devoted commitment with life and through the mingling of our inner and outer experience that the alchemical miracle can occur—the transmutation of the lead in an ordinary human into the gold of a person who expresses the full wisdom, illumination, and potential of his or her authentic nature.

An Invitation to Alchemical Healing

Alchemical Healing combines my knowledge of Chinese medicine and Taoist philosophy with principles and tools drawn from ancient alchemy and modern depth psychology as well as other forms of energy medicine and somatic awareness practices. Through the melding of these various systems, I have crafted an approach to healing that I find well suited to the complex psychospiritual issues my patients face at this time of crisis on the planet.

Alchemical Healing is not a replacement for Western medicine, traditional psychotherapy, or current, more widely accepted ways of practicing Chinese medicine. Rather, it offers a way to touch the subtle body or soul, to help resolve nonphysical forms of human distress, psychic and spiritual imbalances, and longings that are often unresponsive to more conventional techniques. It regards health as a living process you must engage on a daily basis—an ongoing discovery rather than a fixed set of externally imposed rules to follow or something you depend on others to provide. Alchemical Healing may be combined with other forms of medicine or used on its own when the tools of allopathic medicine are not indicated or have already achieved their appropriate goals.

Alchemical Healing is based on the belief that there is a vital force that directs you toward your own growth and fulfillment. This force is an innate, driving, high-grade energy as potent as the physical instincts of survival and reproduction. When this vital force is blocked, ignored, or repressed, illness arises. The goal is not to get you "back to your old self again" but rather for you to discover what you need to change in order to achieve optimal health and a richer, more meaningful life.

Alchemical Healing recognizes the interconnectedness of spirit and matter and honors the value and significance of both these domains, as well as the crucial importance of the connecting link between them: the subtle body or soul. The activated imagination is your most potent tool as you open to working with this level of experience. In the pages of this book, I will describe how to effectively use the concepts and tools of Alchemical Healing. As you work with these ideas, you will learn how to open the door to the alchemical laboratory within you.

The ultimate goal of this kind of healing is a shift in consciousness. When you move from the ordinary perception of everyday life to an expanded alchemical awareness—an illumination that may last a moment or a lifetime—you begin to perceive the purpose, meaning, and beauty of the universe. From this perspective, your life becomes a laboratory where new possibilities arise from challenging symptoms. In this laboratory, you can choose to cultivate the excitement of living on the leading edge of your own growth rather than withdrawing from your suffering. You can exchange your fear of the unknown for curiosity about what's attempting to come to life. Your stuck places, illness, pain, depression, anxiety, and confusion become medicine, bringing with them the potential for you to get closer to, rather than further from, your destiny.

Chapter 2

Repairing a Broken Marriage

Who is there who does not have the fleeting sense—here for a moment and gone again—that once, long ago, we were told a story that now forever eludes us? What was it? Who told it? Why is something known and then not known? Where shall I look for what I have lost? Perhaps we come to realize that if a thing is to be remembered, it has first to be forgotten. The mind had to lose its knowing to the bloodstream in order that there it could be digested, simmered as in a crucible, suffer the sea-change and be given back.

—P. L. Travers, *What the Bee Knows*

Wholeness

Who does not remember a time of wholeness? Perhaps it was that moment just waking from sleep or meeting a lover on a rainy street or hearing the song of crickets in the Summer twilight.

For me, it was when I was very young. My family had just moved to our new house in the country and my parents were head over heels in love—not only with each other but with their garden filled with lilac, mock orange, and roses in the sun; hosta, sweet fern, and lily of the valley in the shadows; and magically, at the center, a lush, full-grown Macoun apple tree.

It was a Sunday in Spring. The three of us were at a nursery, walking along the paths outside the greenhouses. I was in the middle. My father held my left hand, my mother my right. In my memory, the grass was a carpet of emeralds and above our heads the sky opened to an infinite blue that left me breathless with amazement. There were no edges to the world that day as my parents sang out, "One . . . two . . . three . . ." and in effortless unison lifted me by the hands and swung me up into a perfection of flight, my whole body buoyant and filled with happiness.

Although I have had many moments of deep connection, mystical insight, and inspiring beauty since that day, this is my last embodied memory of divine perfection. I treasure it as an affirmation of what I firmly believe as a human and as a healer: despite all appearances to the contrary, each one of us arrives in this world reflecting the integrity, beauty, and perfection of our source.

This source is the original unity that existed before the creation of the universe as well as the undifferentiated chaos that continually generates the new possibilities of the world. Although invisible and ungraspable, source energy animates every aspect of creation. Its power is reflected in the cycles, rhythms, and forms of the natural world. Alchemical traditions from disparate cultures have come up with different ways to name and symbolize this mystery but it is recognized wherever alchemy flourishes. European alchemists called it the "One Thing" or the "quintessence." Egyptian alchemists referred to it with the hieroglyphic *kh*.

Figure 1. Egyptian hieroglyphic *kh*

This hieroglyphic makes up the first letter of the Egyptian word *khem*, which is the root of our word *alchemy*. The hieroglyphic has a dual meaning, on the one hand tangible and material and on the

The Alchemy of Inner Work

other hand intangible and divine. *Kh* is translated as dark soil, referring to the fertile black earth left by the receding tides of the Nile from which all vegetative life emerged. This dark soil was also the source of the metals and precious ores that the early Egyptian alchemists worked with in their laboratories. Alternatively, *kh* is translated as placenta or uterus, the rich inner matrix of the mother's body that shelters and gives life to the developing embryo.

Further, the hieroglyphic *kh* also refers to what alchemists call the "First Matter," a primordial undifferentiated spiritual substance, a chaos, without gender, weight, or form that gives birth to all things and to which all things return. *Kh* is the origin of Heaven and Earth. Endlessly pulsating, creating, and destroying, *kh* is the matrix, the Absolute, and the gateway to the infinite.

Later European alchemists used the symbol of the ouroboros, the mythical serpent who continually devours and emerges from its own being, to graphically express the endlessly regenerating power of the source.

Figure 2. Ouroboros

The ancient Chinese alchemists called it *Tao*. They regarded Tao as the origin of all being, the gate to the essence of everything. From the Taoist as well as from an alchemical perspective, at the beginning and the end of every journey is Tao—this perfect, unknowable wholeness. The Chinese character is a symbol made up of two parts.

Figure 3. Chinese character for *Tao*

Repairing a Broken Marriage

On the right is a picture of a head with a plumed hat. A plumed hat is worn by a leader, a military general, a priest, or a shaman. The feathers on the hat reach up to heaven and bring down the messages of the stars. With guidance from above, the leader begins the journey. On the left is a picture of a foot, indicating a person walking, going somewhere on a path. Without the foot that walks on the Earth, the Way of Heaven cannot be followed.

Tao is the all of you, from the top of your head to the bottom of your feet, from your conscious sun-lit mind to your unconscious lunar instincts. Tao is spirit and matter and all that lies between. The poet Lao Tzu describes it as "The breath that never dies." From this endless breath comes all the living and dying beings and forms of creation. This infinite, formless breathing cannot be known directly and yet you know it through its impression in natural form, its reflection in the world of darkness and light.

Tao eludes the conscious mind but if you quiet the thinking mind for a moment and open the eyes of your heart to your inner world, Tao can be known by the messages of your dreams, your body symptoms, your particular longings and emotions, the impossible coincidences, and strange twists and turns of fate that shape your life. In this way, your small, limited sense of who you are expands until, once again, you are joined with the cosmos.

Living your Tao means living in alignment with your own divine nature. This is the definition of health according to the ancient Chinese. Over the years, I've found that it is also the most accurate definition for me and for the people I work with. Living your Tao has nothing to do with your ordinary ideas about happiness or health. It is not about how much money you make, how beautiful or youthful an appearance you project, or even how long you live. It has to do with whether you are going somewhere, whether you are on your path with your head and feet connected. Living your Tao reflects that you are following the guidance of your inner knowing and not someone else's ideas about who you are supposed to be.

It turns out that following your Tao can look pretty weird from the outside. In fact, "The weirder the better," says Chuang Tzu, one of the greatest Taoist sages of all time. He says to check out that "hunchback catching cicadas with a sticky pole," or that one there with "two toes webbed together and a sixth finger forking off," or that old tree "with trunk distorted, so full of knots, no one can get a straight plank out of it." Strange as these examples may be, Chuang Tzu reminds us that throughout many years of focused practice, the hunchback has come to know the nature of cicadas in and out, and through that has discovered a skill, passion, and singleness of purpose that completely satisfies him. The gnarled tree, which cannot be rounded with a compass or cut with a T-square, has escaped the carpenter's axe and lived for centuries contentedly offering shade and shelter to creatures in the forest. Webbed Toes has stopped trying to be like anyone else and has learned to dance on her own strange feet.

The question is: What is the medicine that ultimately allowed these beings to accept their Tao and become who they were meant to be?

Throughout history, the quest to distill an infinitesimal drop from the source, to gather the primordial power and underlying wholeness of the cosmos, has been the central focus of alchemy. Alchemists regard this distillation as the essential medicine and believe that even a drop would be able to heal the world. As modern-day alchemists, it is our task to discover this source and bring a drop of its healing water back to our ailing world.

The Divine Couple

From One—the Source—Two naturally arises. The arising of Two gives birth to the possibility of polarity. Like the positive and negative poles of a battery create an electrical flow, the space or field that exists between all polarities generates life. Whether you consider the first division of the maternal egg after fertilization, the cracking open of the seed in Spring, or the division of a single sprout into the twin leaves of the dicotyledon, you see that the movement from One to Two is the beginning, the first prerequisite for embodiment and growth. From the divine marriage of these two polar opposites, the world is born and Tao becomes manifest in the infinite forms of creation.

Five thousand years ago, the Taoist sage Fu Hsi recognized the pivotal moment when the two life principles emerged from Tao as the beginning of time. He named these principles *ch'ien*, the creative or spirit power, and *k'un*, the receptive or power of matter. Together, they form the basis of China's greatest alchemical text, The I Ching or Book of Changes. Fu Hsi created two graphic symbols for these two principles:

Ch'ien: Heaven or the Creative

K'un: Earth or the Receptive

The energy of the receptive principle came to be called *yin*. The earliest character was a picture of clouds or something shaded from the sunlight. Over time, the character changed and came to represent the shady side of a hill. Yin represents the principle of matter and the Earth. It is associated with water, coolness, lunar consciousness, inwardness, darkness, and the power of gestation, process, and manifestation. It is also associated with the feminine or uterine aspects of being.

The energy of the active principle came to be called *yang*. The earliest character was a picture of the sun with rays coming down from the sky. Later, the character was redrawn to represent the sunny side of a hill. Yang represents the principle of spirit and Heaven. It is associated with fire, heat, solar consciousness, outwardness, and the power of initiatory impulses. It has also come to be associated with the masculine or phallic aspects of being.

The Alchemy of Inner Work

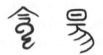

Figure 4. Ancient Chinese graphics for *yin* and *yang*

From the Taoist alchemical perspective, yin and yang are mutually arising and sustaining. They emerge simultaneously from Tao and one cannot exist without the other. Like two partners in a healthy marriage, one is not better, more necessary, or more valuable than the other. Without both partners, the marriage cannot exist.

Like the sunny and shady sides of a hill, yin and yang are not fixed but are relative. As the sun moves from east to west, dawn to dusk, what we know as the yin and yang sides of the hill shift in response to time and the changing position of the sun.

The alchemical notion of Two is beautifully expressed through the *Taiji* symbol, an ancient depiction of yin and yang. This symbol expresses in graphic form the dance of the opposites as they mutually arise from Tao.

Figure 5. *Taiji* or *yin-yang* symbol

The distinguishing feature of the alchemical view is that Two emerges from and retains its connection to One. In his book *The Mystery of Human Relationship*, Nathan Schwartz-Salant writes,

> All of alchemical thinking is concerned with opposites . . .
> Somehow the alchemist had to recognize opposites inherent in
> any process and then to unite them. A spiritual sense of Oneness plays a vital role, for a kind of illumination is often necessary to "see" opposites, an act of discovering order in chaos.

The goal is not for the two principles—spirit and matter, male and female, mind and body, activity and rest—to radically split apart but rather for them to polarize, to separate just enough to come into life-giving relationship.

An imbalance between these two fundamental energies is at the root of many of the psychosomatic and emotional symptoms I treat. I also believe that the severing of connection between these two forces by the dualism of modern consciousness is at the root of many of our most pressing global problems. This split is aggravated for my patients and the planet by our culture's overvaluation of the yang—mind, activity, productivity, speed, expansion, and a more archetypally masculine approach to life—and an undervaluing of the yin—body, rest, idleness, reflection, conservation, cultivation, and the more archetypally feminine approach to life—which has left us devoid of connection to the renewing, gestating, and sustaining power of the inner world.

The Great Divorce

The ancient Chinese understood that the marriage of yin and yang engenders life. Their divorce leads to death. All alchemists share the view that the miracle of life arises from the interplay of these two cosmic polarities and that their separation inevitably leads to a destructive loss of vitality, generativity, and potency. From an alchemical perspective, the separation of these two principles should only be undertaken with the utmost care, for a brief amount of time, and within the safe confines of the alchemical laboratory. Carelessly or unconsciously isolating them from one another will ultimately lead to a dangerous waning of the life force.

However, for the past four hundred years in the Western world, the Cartesian dualistic view of reality has severed the connection between these two polarities. To this day, we create dichotomies that separate yin and yang, matter and spirit, feminine and masculine, the sensing/feeling body and the thinking mind. Spirit has become an abstraction that exists distant from our embodied life, while matter has been relegated to inanimate stuff that can be objectified, used, and discarded without concern for its innate subjectivity.

Today, we see the positive outcome of the great divorce of rationalism in the increase of our capacity to analyze and manipulate the physical world around us. This has led to tremendous gains in the domains of Western science, mechanical engineering, and technology, as well as great strides in the physical aspects of Western medicine, including surgery, diagnostics, and disease prevention and control. When my good friend's son wrapped his car around a tree, we were all deeply grateful for the pinpoint accuracy of the tests and technology, the targeted medications, and the cool, rational minds of the doctors who saved his life.

However, who will be there to support him as he recovers from the shock and emotional trauma of the near-death experience? Who will guide him as he learns how to live a satisfying, self-sustaining, and meaningful life with severe physical limitations? And who will offer him alternatives to alcohol and opioids as he grapples with the chronic pain resulting from his injuries? In the words of my doctor friend, it is important to know what our different kinds of medicine are meant to do.

Despite all the gains of our mastery of the physical world, there have been losses in the domain of human spiritual and psychological well-being as the nonphysical aspects of our lives have been increasingly marginalized and denied. In addition, the splitting off of matter from its "other"—the spiritual essence of life—has led to a lack of respect for the innate divinity of the natural world. As a result, human beings have come to regard nature, as well as their own bodies, as commodities, products to be bought and sold for profit, stuff to be manipulated solely for human gain. The outcome of this divorce is a culture that is unwell and a planet that is seriously threatened.

Given the intricate complexity of the issues currently confronting humanity, black and white thinking no longer offers adequate solutions. We are faced with the crucial question of how to repair the marriage of these severed cosmic principals—in our own being as well as in the world around us.

The Cracking

My father developed a brain tumor when I was ten years old, and my sun-lit world came crashing down in pieces. Although it had been many years since my early experience of original divine wholeness, I had remained a kind of magical child, closely connected to my own imagination and the nonhuman world of plants and animals. The shock of my father's illness was the final death blow to my childhood, the cracking apart of my original integrity.

I felt lost, alone, and responsible for alleviating my father's suffering. I had no way to understand this experience in relationship to the rest of my life. When I look back, I realize that the worst of it was not my father's illness but rather my family's response to his illness. My parents did not talk about it with me. I had no idea if my father would live or die. I was left alone to deal with my own fear, grief, and all the unnamed and unspoken emotions rushing through my home.

I responded by going numb, putting on a mask, and acting "as if." I pretended I was okay in order not to be a bother to anyone. I now know that there are names for what happened to me. Western psychologists call it dissociation, by which they mean a detachment from reality as a way to cope with an overwhelming experience. Chinese physicians call it a *shen* disturbance, by which they mean that a person's shen or spirit separates from the physical body in order to protect itself in the face of shock or trauma. Alchemists call it the cracking of the vessel, an event that is inevitably followed by a *nigredo*, a darkening, dissolution, or depression that is an essential phase of an alchemical process of transformation.

For me, that darkening was a depression and withdrawal from relatedness, ambition, and my own creative fire that lasted throughout my adolescence and well into my adulthood. What I eventually came to understand is that from an alchemical perspective, the cracking of the vessel and the subsequent nigredo is actually a moment of great potential. It is the first step on the journey, the beginning of the Great Work of embracing embodiment as a means of remembering and reclaiming our wholeness, our Tao.

Alchemists have always held to a different view of embodiment than that of mainstream Judeo-Christian religious doctrine. They do not accept the idea that matter and spirit are separate, or that transcendence of the body is the ultimate goal of spiritual development. They reject the denigration of the body that began with Plato's argument:

> The body is a source of endless trouble to us . . . and is liable also to diseases which overtake and impede us in the search after true being; it fills us full of loves, and lusts, and fears, and fancies of all kinds, and endless foolery, and . . . takes away from us the power of thinking at all.

To alchemists, the yin domain of earth, matter, and the body is the laboratory where our spiritual work gets done. Without the containment, resistances, and often frustrating challenge of embodiment, transformation is impossible.

I see now that the early traumatic experience of my father's brain tumor, the numbness that followed, and the amnesia around my own divine wholeness was the beginning of an unfolding process. I believe that my choice to become an acupuncturist and healer was an expression of my Tao. But more importantly, that inherent nature was born in response to a need to heal from my own wounding. As I've healed, I've come to help others learn to respond differently to illness and the inevitable sufferings and challenges of embodied life. My attitude toward healing is shaped by what I lived through in my own family but also by the alchemical idea that the parts of life you resist, the painful experiences you reject or deny, the parts of yourself you hate or are ashamed of, are actually points of growth, places where your soul is invited to incarnate more fully.

It took many years, the help of many gifted teachers, and long practice with the tools I am presenting in this book to bring me back to the place where I began, so that my early memory of wholeness could be, in the words of author and mythologist P. L. Travers, "[d]igested, simmered as in a crucible, suffer the sea-change and be given back."

Healing as a Return to Wholeness

If you consider the root of the English word *health*, you find there is an ancient, implicit understanding about the purpose of the healing process embedded in alchemical ideas and principles. The word *health* comes from the Anglo Saxon *hal*, which is also the root of the words *heal* and *whole*. In addition, *hal* is the etymological ancestor of the word *holy*. From this perspective, healing is much more than fixing the cracks in something broken so it can work the way it did before. Instead, healing is a process that brings a new, more inclusive and efficient wholeness to a living system that has fragmented, a system that has lost its integrity, its purpose, and its vital connection to the divine.

This same connection between healing and wholeness is found in the Chinese character *hé*, which forms part of the word *yùhé*, to heal or to cure. Hé is a picture of a lid fitting perfectly over the top of an opening. Hé implies the idea of coming together, the combining of parts that result in a safely closed container or wholeness.

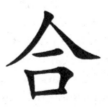

Figure 6. *Hé*, the Chinese character used in the word *yùhé*,
to heal or to cure

The roots of these words reveal that the archetypal concern of the healing process is not alleviating suffering but rather bringing parts back together and mending the brokenness that is the source of suffering. Healing, at its root, is the path that returns you to wholeness and brings you back to your innate and imperative relationship to your source. Healing is a return to the holiness that is your origin.

Chapter 3

The Connecting Link of Imagination and the Soul

Separate the Earth from Fire, the Subtle from the Gross, gently and with great Ingenuity.

It rises from Earth to Heaven and descends again to Earth, thereby combining within Itself the powers of both the Above and the Below.

—The Emerald Tablet (Precept Four)

Coyote Song

I heard her sing many times before she showed up in my treatment room. I knew her voice before I knew her—hard to define, yet distinct and unforgettable. When I saw her perform at local gatherings, I was struck by the sweatshirt she wore with the hood pulled down to hide her eyes, her voice emerging from the dark moon circle under the cowl. Like a monk at compline, she sang from the night, without revealing her facial markers of individual identity.

Michaela's email arrived out of the blue, like a calling card from the forest. "I would love to make an appointment to work with you. I'm in a very stuck place psychologically and physically and I recognize that I need a routine of healing work. Others have told me how helpful you've been, and I have thought of you many times."

I was honored but also surprised that I had entered her orb of awareness. I was cautious in my reply, sensing that she might flee back to the forest if I didn't stay deep in my listening, if I didn't pay close attention to the nearly inaudible cues.

She arrived exactly on time for the first session, a strikingly beautiful woman in her late twenties with a bit of adolescent wildness about her. Even though she had no hood pulled over her eyes, I couldn't quite get a read on her. Her face never settled down, but instead changed constantly as if there were several different possibilities in each moment of encounter. When she sat across from me, she looked away and seemed almost apologetic about being so punctual. "I show up when I want to but other times I disappear," she told me. "No one knows where I am. I hide out."

Her presenting issues: periods of deep depression and withdrawal, extreme sensitivity to people and their feelings, a lack of psychic boundary, anxiety about things under the surface, and terrible bouts of jealousy and anger.

She said,

> I know I have a gift, but I don't know who I am, what I want to do with my life. I end up being how other people want me to be and then I rebel, get mad deep down, withdraw, and turn myself into an emotional knot. I know I can heal people with my voice. But I sabotage myself with bad habits and waste my time worrying and being taken over by jealousy. At times I completely lose it over stories that aren't even real that I make up about my boyfriend. Or, when I am in one of my depressed states, I turn into a hermit. I can't go out. I don't like myself. I hate the way I look. I don't want people to see me.

Our work began with conversation. What were her goals?

> I want to be fully present, comfortable with people, part of a community. I want to stop wandering from place to place, living with my boyfriend or out of my car. I want to develop some routines that keep me on track and away from my bad habits. I want a sense of purpose, a way to find a way to take my music seriously, to use my gift.

In addition to talking, we worked with acupuncture, flower essences, essential oils, and meditation exercises. I listened intently not only to her words but also to the messages of her gestures and the intonations in her voice. She also started to pay attention to her dreams. She liked the treatments, especially the flower essences. She noticed that her moods were brighter and a bit more stable. She was getting out with friends, singing more.

I reflected back to her that despite her stated view of herself as someone who disappears, has no purpose, and can't follow through, I experienced her as being very committed to our work together, punctual, responsible about payment, remembering to take the remedies I made for her, and exploring my suggestions for work between sessions. Again, she gave me that rueful look, as if she were hesitant to admit her own curiosity, hunger, and determined strength, her deep desire to know herself, and her excitement about the possibility of bringing her full power to the world. "Oh, yes," she said, "I can show up when I want to."

A few months after we began working together, she was invited to sing at a Summer festival in the hills of northern New Hampshire. Through a long evening she would sing to the people gathered and her voice would carry them across midnight into the early morning. She was shy, uncertain about whether she was up to the task. But after some gentle coaxing and then some more emphatic demands from the festival organizers, she agreed.

I saw her the day before she left for the festival. "I'm ready," she said. "I'm taking the remedies you gave me and I like them. I do feel afraid, afraid that I won't be able to do it. But I'm doing it anyway." She turned and half-smiled as she left, looking back once before gliding out the door.

I wasn't at the festival, but what I heard from others and what I know was that her voice came out of the dark night and wove a spell over the whole gathering. The waning gibbous moon rose with her voice and traversed the sky as she sang. And somewhere in the middle of the moon's course, the coyotes arrived. At first, she was too much a part of her own sound to notice their presence. But then the harmonies began. Her notes disappeared into the night, then returned, deepened, layered, transformed by the fur-coated wily tricksters of the forest.

"Suddenly, I heard them. I knew they were there. All around me. They were singing with me. I joined with them. We became one song. I couldn't see their faces, but I felt them in the darkness. I forgot myself completely. I sang in a way I've never sung before."

As I sat listening to her story, I saw her face coming into focus for the first time. Sensitive, elegant, alert to every nuance of sound. And next to her, behind her, I saw the animals watching, listening, cautious and brilliantly acute in their awareness, sniffing out safe and unsafe, tracking me closely.

"The coyotes," I offered. "They are still with you."

"Yes, I know, and I think they always will be," she answered.

As we both admitted to seeing the unseeable, something shifted; not completely, not forever, but for that one moment, which was also an eternity. I knew we had moved to a new level in our work.

"The coyotes," I asked, "What do you know about them?"

"They come and go. They are tricky. You have to be careful not to be fooled by them. They can lead you down the wrong path, like drinking or getting involved with the wrong people," she answered. I knew she was telling me something important about herself.

"But what if you turn that around?" I asked. And I saw the coyotes around her perking up their ears, sniffing the air, alert to some intrigue. She gave me the familiar grin, as if she knew more than she would say. "What if instead of seeing their trickiness, their coming and going as a problem, you see it as a power they give you. They are survivors. They know what's safe and unsafe. They can sniff out danger as well as sustenance. They intuit when they need to go back into the forest to rest, to gather up their strength, to learn new songs. What if that was also something true about you?"

She took a long, deep breath. The coyotes lifted their heads and their noses twitched. I knew she knew, and they knew. I had seen her. And she, for a moment, had also seen herself. She looked at me and started to laugh. "Oh, I get it," she said. "That's different."

Then the coyotes stretched and yawned and relaxed lazily on the rug. She lay down on the treatment table, closed her eyes, and

The Alchemy of Inner Work

rested. I needled the acupuncture point called Palace of Weariness—
the palace where the wild, the hunted, the lost, and wounded come
to heal.

In our work together, Michaela and I had slipped through the
gate of ordinary reality and entered a different domain of awareness. In this place, our habitual ways of organizing the world shifted.
The distinctions we ordinarily make between inner and outer, self
and other, human and nonhuman dissolved momentarily. We knew
beyond the accepted boundaries of individual identity, beyond the
limits of universally verifiable fact. We perceived things we could
not perceive with our everyday senses alone. We gathered and wove
together the threads of reality in a new way, allowing the gifts of
intuition, imagination, and spirit to be part of the tapestry. In the
words of the ancient Chinese healers, "We saw what cannot be seen
with the ordinary eyes, heard what cannot be heard with the ordinary ears. . . knew what only the heart can know." We touched what
is sometimes called "the subtle body." We entered the inner laboratory of alchemy and began a process of Alchemical Healing.

The Subtle Body

The concept of an invisible but palpable energy body that lives
alongside our physical structure conflicts with the scientific view of
the body as a mechanical, biochemical system. The mutable nature
of this "other body," its tendency to shy away from the light of the
rational mind and the fact that it can't be weighed, measured, or
pinned down makes it difficult to talk about in ordinary language.
Yet, this other immaterial body has been a central concern of philosophers, healers, and spiritual seekers in Eastern and Western cultures
for at least the past 2,500 years.

In my years of experience, I've found that there is no way to
work effectively at a psycho-spiritual level with acupuncture points,
flower essences, astrology, dreams, or any other alchemical modal-
ity without an understanding of this aspect of our being. Despite
the challenges it presents to language and the rational mind, it has
been essential for me to find a way to conceptualize, talk about, and

consciously work with the subtle body. I believe that the recognition and recovery of the subtle body is a prerequisite if we are to move forward with the development of a new approach to healing.

When you receive an acupuncture treatment, consult a trained astrologer, take flower essences, or attend a yoga class, you are touched and moved in a way that exists outside the parameters of what can be proven, measured, or analyzed. These modalities work on a part of you that is not purely physical. For example, a good yoga teacher will emphasize that the benefit of pigeon pose is not just the deep stretch it offers to the external rotators of your hip but also the opening it creates for you to stretch into a deeper knowing that you can let go and trust. The challenge of the asana invites you into a relationship with your own assumptions and resistances as well as your strengths. As you hold the pose, you learn to quiet your mind and listen more closely to the underlying stream of energy moving through you. While any yoga class will exercise your physical body in obvious ways, a really satisfying class will touch something that results in you leaving in a profoundly different mental/emotional state than when you went in.

Of course, this sense of well-being is reflected in measurable changes to your physical body, including shifts in heart rate, hormone levels, and brain wave patterns. But an alchemist would say that through the postures, the breathing practices, the visualizations, and the chanting, you went through a process of inner transformation. The yogi would say that you balanced your chakras and moved your prana. The acupuncturist would say that you cleared a blockage in your meridians and enlivened your *qi*. The Kabbalist would say that you aligned your ten energy spheres and made contact with your inner angels.

Who is right? How can these systems with their very different filters, maps, and technologies all refer to the same phenomenon? How can they all work? The unifying factor of all these systems is that they work at the level of the alchemical subtle body.

The word *subtle* comes from the Latin *subtilis*, which means "fine, thin, delicate, finely woven." The prefix *sub* means "under" and the stem *tilis*, from *tela* means "web, net, warp of fabric." The word refers to a delicate fabric of the finest thread. A related meaning refers to a person with the capacity for refinement of thought, insight, and perception. And less commonly but still relevant to this investigation, the term is also sometimes used to describe a person of sly, tricky, crafty, and artful character.

A related idea is found in the ancient Indian myth of Indra's net. This tale describes the universe as a magical net that the god Indra hangs over his palace on Mount Meru, the center of the cosmos. Indra's net has a multifaceted jewel at each vertex, and each jewel is reflected in all of the other jewels. The net is a metaphorical description of the Buddhist concept of interpenetration of all things, and symbolically describes how this interpenetration and mutual relatedness of parts is a primary truth of the cosmos.

These clues reveal that thread and the weaving of thread are universally recognized ways of describing this background matrix of life. Also implicit are qualities of uncertainty, craft, fineness of texture, and interconnectedness. These roots describe the subtle body as something that is woven. It is a finely textured tissue, nearly imperceptible to the ordinary senses, vaporous yet tensile, even tricky and deceptive at times in its presentation. In *The Doctrine of the Subtle Body*, the alchemist G. R. S. Mead writes:

> It must, however, be always clearly understood that, for our philosophers, spirit . . . is the subtle body, an embodiment of a finer order of matter than that known to physical sense, and not soul proper. By body, moreover, is not meant developed and organized form, but rather "essence" or "plasm" that may be graded, or as it were woven into various textures. In itself unshaped, it is capable of receiving the impression or pattern of any organized form.

The grading, morphing tendency that Mead remarks on as well as its capacity to be impressed, patterned, and woven explains why the subtle body can change its presentation depending on culture, time, and the systems brought to bear on its perception.

In Chinese medicine, the subtle body is impressed with the pattern of the acupuncture meridians and points, the Five Elements and the Five Spirits. In Vedic yoga, it takes the shape of the energy centers and channels called the chakras and *nadis;* in the Kabbalistic tradition, it forms the sephirot of the Tree of Life. In astrology, the subtle body is shaped by the planetary movements against a backdrop of starry constellations. In Western archetypal psychology, it flows into the patterns of dreams, gods, and goddesses and other mythical symbols. Although these various alchemical systems have outer differences, they all recognize the presence of a pattern underlying the manifest world, a formless chaos of primal threads that is ordered to form psychically activated mystical shapes, designs, maps, and symbols, which ultimately make meaningful correspondences to human life. These varied expressions of subtle body are the foundation of all methodologies that support human psycho-spiritual development.

Weaving happens on a loom where there is an overlapping of horizontal and vertical threads. This overlap of warp and weft where two opposites meet and join is necessary in order to form a durable, unified fabric. From this association, I have come to see that the subtle body is formed by a process of weaving—a linking together of two polarities—matter and spirit, yin and yang, self and other. The subtle body brings opposites together in new ways, it unifies parts that have been separated.

Using a different metaphor, I liken the web of the subtle body to the energized electro-magnetic field that forms between the opposing north and south poles of a magnet. However, unlike the field that is created by moving electrically charged particles, the field of the subtle body pulses with psychic energy expressed as awareness or consciousness. The subtle body vibrates with vital, animating breaths of life rather than a measurable physical force. While the electro-magnetic force field powers electrical and mechanical systems, the field of the subtle body powers the life force that gets you out of bed in the morning. It is a psychic rather than a physical phenomenon, so the subtle body is qualitative rather than quantitative. Western science cannot measure subtle-body effects; it exists outside and beyond the evaluating obsession of the current dominant worldview. For this reason, Western medicine and science have for the most part ignored or actively denied this expression of human experience.

Despite the fact that it cannot be quantified, the subtle body has qualities, effects, and initiating tendencies that affect us at unconscious levels and can even be consciously perceived when we use our senses in a heightened way. For example, when I first met Benjamin at a Body Sacred retreat, something invisible but very real came to life in the field between us. This "something" was tricky, elusive, and powerful. It drew us together and then kept bringing us back into connection even when we tried to separate. Over the years, this "something" has directed our life in many unexpected ways. These kinds of psychic field events happen all the time. You meet a new person and immediately feel a strong click or an equally palpable aversion. It can't be measured but you know it's real. You pick up these bits of information even if you can't precisely see where they are coming from. For example, you walk into a house where someone recently died and you're filled with an inexplicable heaviness. Or you walk through an old growth forest and feel a rain of blessing, some kind of love opening your heart.

For modern Westerners, our inability to capture or analyze the substance that makes up the subtle body means we must take a leap of faith when we attempt to relate to this quality of experience. You must embrace a kind of knowing that is beyond reason or external verification. You must find a way to trust the subtle body's trickiness, its mutability, its crafty uncertainty. Alchemists call it "Mercurius," quicksilver, that wizened face peeking out from the bark of an old tree, the scent of the moon at midnight, clouds quilting the western mountains, honey pouring from green leaves, the living world caught for just a moment and then gone.

As an alchemist, you will consciously develop this way of perceiving the world while maintaining your capacity for critical thinking and careful observation. You will open to a part of your being that has been largely dormant, to some degree even atrophied. You will revive and re-invigorate a psychic muscle every person is born with and rediscover your innate ability to discern the outer world not only with your ordinary senses but also through a subtler form of awareness that I call "the imaginal."

No one can tell you if the images you see are real. As an alchemist you determine the value as well as the validity of your subtle body's experience. This experience can be uncomfortable living as we do in a culture that insists on external benchmarks as affirmation for what is valid. Michaela's and my recognition of her coyote companions shifted her life in a profoundly meaningful way. Likewise, your emotional, psychological, and spiritual responses are your guide. Pay attention to your inner vitality, your self-understanding, your growth, and the changes in your outer relationships. This is the work. This is the laboratory.

Soul

Often when I teach about the subtle body, people ask if it is the same as the soul. It is not. The subtle body is the finely textured cloth we weave with our awareness, caring, craft, intention, and perhaps, most importantly, our imagination to give the soul a skin that can be seen and touched. Developing our skill as a weaver and the special kind of sight we need to see the threads is the work of alchemy. The many alchemical maps and technologies that have evolved through time create a wardrobe; garments we drape over the infinite that allow us to make contact with the soul within the confines of a physical reality.

In earlier times, shamans, alchemists, and the indigenous people of all cultures lived in close relationship with this elusive, immaterial other. They tended to the web of connection on a daily basis through song, story, ritual, and prayer. So once again, I turn back to ancient times, to the indigenous roots of our language as well as the ancient symbols, stories, and myths to find more clues about the subtle body and the soul.

The English word *soul* comes from the early Celts who were fisherfolk and farmers. Soul is related to their word *sele*, which means sea. For these people, who woke in the dim glow of first morning to row their boats into the mist in search of salmon, mackerel, smelt, and eels, the soul is a shadow that rises up from the deep waters. It gives life but also takes life away. Drowning in sele's unfathomable depths was an ever-present fear for the Celts but equally present was the possibility of pulling up treasures—shimmering pearls, spiraling nautilus shells, golden coins—amidst the wriggling silver chaos of fish pulled from their nets.

One of the soul's most potent images is found in the story of the Selkie, told by the Celts, Scots, Icelanders, Siberians, and all the way across the Bering Strait by the native people of the American Northwest. The Selkie is a magical seal who comes up from the ocean depths, removes her outer pelt (her seal/soul skin), and turns into a shimmering milky skinned woman who dances in the moonlight on warm Summer nights. One evening, a fisherman comes upon her dancing on a rock rising up from the water. He is dazzled by her beauty and vows to make her his bride. Night after Summer night, he rows out to watch as she removes her pelt, dances, then puts her skin back on and returns to her home in the sea.

One night, he manages to steal her water skin while she is dancing. Without her seal skin, she is trapped in human form and cannot return to her true home. She reluctantly leaves the sea to live on land, becomes the fisherman's wife, and bears his half-seal, half-human child. She comes to love her husband and her son, but gradually, after years on land, her unprotected flesh becomes dry, her nails crack, her glorious hair falls out strand by strand, and her glittering, liquid dark eyes become so dim she can no longer see the moonlight.

Year after year, she waits patiently for her husband to return her skin and set her free, but he loves her too much and cannot bear to lose her. After seven long years on shore, she goes off in search of her skin. Beneath a stone at the edge of the ocean cliffs, she finds it where her husband hid it all those years ago. She dresses herself and swims away in the night, back to her home in the sea.

But before she swims away, she sings out to her son,

I leave but I am always with you. Only touch what I have touched, my knife, my stone carvings, the sticks I rubbed together to make our fires and you will feel me near. Listen

The Connecting Link of Imagination and the Soul   **37** carefully to the sounds of the sea and I will whisper my secrets in your ear. Remember me and I will always remember you and you will know my magic.

Her son becomes a carver of stone, a famous storyteller, and healer, and people come from far and wide to learn the secrets of the soul from him.

This story has helped me understand my own experience. What I have learned is that if I try to catch the soul, illuminate it, and keep it too long on land, it will become dry and brittle. It will lose its healing magic. But if I go to the edge of the sea, my night vision activated, be still and wait, the soul will rise up from the depths and come to meet me.

The Imagination

Imagination is an intrinsic part of our humanity and our bridge to the land of the soul. It gives us the ability to form inner images of things that are not present to our ordinary senses. The imagination has been problematic for Western philosophers since Aristotle likened it to fantasy and declared that, unlike the intellect, it is one of our faculties that "is not always correct." Western philosophy, religion, and science have followed in Aristotle's footsteps and remained suspicious of the imagination.

In contrast, ancient alchemists aligned with artists and mystics to view the imagination as sacred, serving as a connecting link between the human and divine worlds. They believed that through our capacity to meditate, dream, and imagine, we access enlivening forces and formative powers that are not apparent to our rational minds and conscious awareness. This inborn capacity to perceive the spiritual domain and transcend the limitations of our ordinary senses allows us to communicate with divine realms, perceive the subtle body, and begin to bring to life our entelechy, the fulfillment of our spiritual potential.

Taoist alchemists regarded the imagination as the domain of the *hun* or cloud soul, the yang spirit whose job is to bring the messages of the celestial bodies—the sun, moon, and stars—down to

Earth. The sixteenth-century European alchemist Martin Ruland the Younger spoke of the imagination in his *Lexicon of Alchemy* as "[t]he star in man, the celestial or supercelestial body." C. G. Jung points out that Ruland's definition firmly connects the imagination to the divine in us, what Paracelsus called the alchemical *astrum*, or sacred essence of life. This special kind of heavenly luminosity opens us to our star map and our destiny. Jung took this one step further to describe the imagination as a "[c]oncentrated extract of the life force, both physical and psychic."

The word *imagination*, which comes from the Latin *imaginatio*, refers to the real and literal human power to craft images and create symbols. Writes Jung,

> Imaginatio is the active evocation of inner images . . . an authentic feat of thought or ideation, which does not spin aimless and groundless fantasies "into the blue"—does not, that is to say, just play with its objects, but tries to grasp the inner facts and portray them in images true to their nature. This activity is an *opus*, a work.

In fact, it is the work of alchemy and it is directly linked to the weaving of the subtle body and the clothing of the soul.

Imagination contains the root word *magus*. Through magus, imagination joins the word group correlating to "make, machine, and might" and from there back to the ancient Indo-European root *mag(h)*, which is also related to the word *magic*. The magician or magi is one who makes, creates, crafts, and in particular, makes a thing into something new. The magician works with matter and sleight of hand, transforms and recreates the world through the clever, tricky, and skillful use of the imagination.

Essential to magic and to imaginative processes are the qualities of ingenuity, uncertainty, daring, elegance, and most importantly, creativity. Magic asks that you suspend disbelief and discover the determination to see the world differently. These are also important characteristics of alchemy and Alchemical Healing, for without imagination it is impossible to see the subtle body or to truly touch the soul.

Continuing the Journey

Several weeks after the coyotes arrived, Michaela did not show up for her appointment. I waited fifteen minutes, twenty, half an hour, and then gave up. She had never been even five minutes late.

I began to worry. Voices started in my head. I was on the wrong track. I'd frightened her off, missed important cues. She'd flown away, back to the forest. Disappeared again under her dark cowl, into her depressed withdrawn despair. The voices escalated. "Who do you think you are? You're kidding yourself that the other world matters, that it's a space that can heal. Nothing has changed as a result of your meeting with the coyotes."

"How dare you trust in this world that has no existence," a particularly denigrating voice snarled at me.

I left the office and went for a walk in the woods. I sat by a pond and watched the sunlight and water play with the images of trees and stones. I felt the pond's presence as a sweet forgiveness. When I returned to my office, there was a phone message from Michaela followed by an email:

> Dear Lorie,
>
> I had the wildest morning, which led to missing your appointment—and frantically trying to find a way to call to let you know, which I am so sorry didn't happen until too late! I am really sorry for missing the appointment and I do plan on paying for that. I don't take the appointments lightly and I would love to schedule another appointment with you. Meanwhile, I'm noticing an amazing shift in how I'm showing up to my life . . . there's so much work to do but I'm just incredibly amazed at how gently yet strongly you have helped me begin this work.
> Michaela

And so, we will continue, Michaela and I, and a small pack of wild coyotes and who knows who else will show up along the way. The journey will not be brief or easy and the path will often be unclear. Depression, anxiety, and uncertainty of purpose are not "cured" in a few sessions. Identity, meaning, relationship, and intention all take time to crystallize. Michaela will have other bouts of depression and withdrawal. But we turned a corner. Michaela's soul came out from under her cloak of darkness and, for just a moment, let me see her face.

After all, you'll find there is a crafty, tricky quality to the soul and to the world of the subtle body. In this world, images appear and disappear. Things are not always what they seem. Quite suddenly, the parameters of time and space dissolve into their background matrix of infinity. Where you thought you caught a glimpse of a lifting veil, darkness returns. Despite its mercurial tendency, its ephemeral and shifting nature, its urge to hide and seek and play tricks with your mind, the soul ultimately wants to be seen, related to, cared for, and loved. This is the secret. This witnessing is what welcomes spirit back to matter and transforms lead into gold.

Chapter 4

The Alchemical Quest

When you don't follow your nature there is a hole in the universe where you were supposed to be.

—Dane Rudhyar, *Person Centered Astrology*

Beginning with Starlight

Many years ago, on a day that feels like yesterday, on a brand-new leafy morning in early Spring, quite suddenly the ground beneath my feet shifted. Drawn down by unseen hands, I sat on the earth and took a great gulp of air. I placed my fingers on my belly, on the field of blood-red living stone at the center of my being and felt something happen.

At that very moment, a spark of fire exploded in my womb. The cosmos tipped and one single, unique speck of starlight fell from the infinite chaotic void of heaven to pierce my body. As that single flash began to unfurl into a tiny galaxy within me, I transformed from maiden to mother.

I knew that morning. I had no doubt. But it was another two weeks before the slip of paper pronounced me pregnant. As my body began to change, my psyche also shifted. "I" was no longer just me. I was the carrier of another consciousness.

My daughter Nina was born nine months later at 7:27 p.m. on the Winter solstice as her father and I lit the seventh candle, the eternal miraculous flame of Chanukah. The midwife swaddled her in a blanket and handed her to me to hold in my arms for the first time. When she looked up at me—as she oriented herself to a new world of breath, body, temperature, and touch—I saw the sparkle of that unique speck of starlight shining back at me from the glimmering infinity of her eyes.

Twenty-three years later, my daughter had grown into a young woman and my mother was dying. For days, my mother had been talking about finding a way out of her body. She spoke about a point at the top of her head that she imagined she could fly through as she embarked on what she viewed as her soul's next adventure. Over and over, she asked us to repeat the prayer from the *Tibetan Book of the Dead* that speaks of "[e]jecting one's consciousness into the space of the unborn Rigpa," the phrase Tibetan adepts use to describe the transfer of awareness from the limitations of incarnation to the vast expanse of the universal mind. Sometimes in my mother's dreamy half-sleep states she would tell us that she was waiting for "[t]hat Karl von Rigpa to come with his special car."

"I need that car," she told us, the car that would carry her off to the wide flower fields of heaven. Then she would laugh, recognizing that she was in a slightly delusional state and ask me to "[n]eedle that point again . . . the one at the top of my head . . . the one that opens the doorway."

On a cold Winter night in December, nine days after her ninety-eighth birthday, nearly a century after her unique speck of starlight dropped down into my grandmother's womb, Benjamin, Nina, and I watched as my mother's spirit left her body. Outside there was a dusting of snow on the ground. Inside, a warm fire glowed in the wood stove. On the windowsill beside my mother's bed was a bowl of white roses.

I felt a breath as my mother's spirit flew up into the spaciousness of the night. Then the brightness left her eyes and she was gone. Somewhere beyond the house, the night, the darkness, I saw her standing on a rock by the edge of the sea. She spread her wings and lifted back into the stars.

While researching information for my first book, I came across a Taoist story that puts into words what I experienced at the first glimmer of my daughter's becoming and the last gleam of my mother's being.

According to this tale, at the moment of conception an unseen hand takes hold of the Big Dipper, dips the ladle down into the Milky Way, and scoops up light from the river of stars. As the sperm penetrates the ovum and a single egg divides in two, the ladle pours a speck of starlight from heaven down into the mother's womb. The spot where the starlight penetrates the ovum ultimately becomes the vertex of the head and a point called One Hundred Meetings. It is said that this starlight directs the organizing of form from the matrix of a mother's essences. As the egg transforms into embryo into fetus and then child—from our first to last incarnate moment—this speck of illumination remains with us. During life, it resides in our hearts. At death, it releases through the point at the top of the head and returns to its home in the heavens.

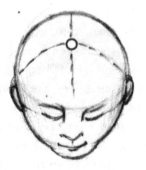

Figure 7. Acupuncture point: One Hundred Meetings

European alchemists called this speck of brilliance that arrives and returns through the point of One Hundred Meetings the *scintilla.* Kabbalists call it *obr.* Taoists call it *shen*, which is most often translated as *spirit.*

When we experience serious shock, trauma, or loss, this light may also leave temporarily through the doorway of One Hundred Meetings. The absence of the spirit leads to what the Chinese call a shen disturbance. While the shen is gone, you will feel disoriented and confused about who you are or where you are going. Sometimes people live for many years or a lifetime with the shen partially absent, in an ongoing state of shen disturbance. The task of Alchemical Healing is to invite this spirit back to its nest in the heart.

Unlike our modern notion of spirit, shen was not an abstraction for ancient Chinese physicians. Even for modern acupuncturists, shen is something we can learn to perceive. You see it in the eyes of a healthy child as well as those of a wise old sage. You feel it when you connect to other beings through relatedness and love. You glimpse it in flashes of intuition, moments of inspiration, when suddenly the path clears, and you know what you need to do next. I feel it as a sense of presence when a previously upset or distracted patient gets up from the treatment table after a session, looks directly at me, smiles, and says, "I'm back."

Once, after needling One Hundred Meetings, a photographer patient said, "I feel like I can see again!" After a pause, he added, "I don't know why it's taken me so long to figure this out, but I just got it. The reason I've been so confused, tired, and dulled out . . . I need to do more than just shoot for advertising campaigns. I need to get back to taking pictures of things I care about. I need to remember why I became a photographer." Soon after, he rescheduled an appointment because he was heading off to document a hurricane. The text he sent to me read, "Yep, I'm going back to what I love. Making films and meeting new people. Bless up!"

Shen is a star seed—a speck of spirit—that drops down into the world of matter where it can take root, sprout, grow, and blossom. It is the very first inkling of consciousness and the last flicker of awareness. It will guide you along the path of your Tao on Earth and then take you back to your source in the stars when your life is over. It is the luminosity of your authentic nature. It is the answer, "I am" to the question, "Who Am I?"

The Self

The powerful initiating, activating, and organizing quality of spirit is at the heart of all alchemical systems. Today, the good news is that studies of spirituality's role in healing are finding a place in many medical school curricula, yet for the past four hundred years spirit has played an insignificant role in modern Western science and medicine. In keeping with his scientific orientation, Sigmund Freud, considered to be the father of modern psychology, did not recognize the significance of spirit in a healthy human life, nor did most of his followers. However, in the early years of the twentieth century, Freud's renegade student, psychiatrist and psychic explorer C. G. Jung, came across the concept of an inner spiritual light innate to all human beings in his studies of Eastern philosophy. The idea captivated him and helped him to understand things he was observing in his own personal inner process as well as in his clinical work with patients.

Jung observed that as people delved into their own unconscious, learned to listen to their dreams, and trusted the wisdom of their imagination as well as the perplexing obsessions, body symptoms, coincidences, and apparent accidents that brought them into analysis, they discovered a kind of inner guidance that gave a new orientation to their life. Although this inner guidance did not always direct people in ways that made sense or were in keeping with conventional attitudes and values, it always led them in a direction of healing, vitality, and an increase in integrity with their own inner truth, which in turn fostered their creative engagement with the world around them. As Jung researched further into ancient Eastern and Western texts, he found that what he was witnessing in his patients—this phenomenon of an inner guidance and organizing principle—wasn't a new concept. It was something that was recognized and documented by alchemists and mystics over thousands of years.

The idea of a Self that connects with and emanates the light of spirit became the defining focus and hallmark of Jung's work and the psychology he developed throughout his lifetime. In fact, Jung's final, definitive severing of his connection to Freud was caused by his belief that a spiritual impulse to manifest the Self rather than the physical instinct to procreate and survive is the central driving force of a human life.

The work of Alchemical Healing follows in the footsteps of the ancient mystics and alchemists as well as the radical position of C. G. Jung. This work begins with the foundational premise that just as the gravitational pull of the sun at the center of the solar system keeps the Earth in orbit, there is a radiant Self at the center of your being that organizes the unfolding of your life. The challenges and obstacles of embodied life may temporarily dim this light, but they can also shift your life into greater alignment. It all depends on how you respond to these difficulties. From the perspective of Alchemical Healing, the work of aligning your life choices and actions with this guiding energy is the key to realizing health.

Entelechy

Eastern and Western esoteric philosophy, alchemical traditions, and depth psychology all recognize an innate, inborn goal-directed spiritual impulse in human beings that is separate from, yet related to, the instincts of the physical body. This impulse calls you toward the fullest possible expression of your being, urging you to come as close as possible to an identity that expresses the Self.

The alchemical attitude insists that every living being has this speck of guiding divinity hidden within. The word that comes closest to expressing this idea comes from the Greek *entelechy*. The word is made up of two parts: the first part, *en*, means "to have," the second, *telos*, means "completion." Entelechy suggests that my beginning also contains my end. It means that life has an innate, inborn purpose and direction. From the perspective of entelechy, spirit infuses form and matter with divine intention. Consciousness is going somewhere, and you too have a destiny, an implicit wholeness and completion already in you at the moment of your birth.

Entelechy tells us that the acorn holds the oak in its thumb-sized shell and the lead already knows its gold. Each and every one of your trillions of cells carries genetic material imprinted with the potential of who you are truly meant to be. This knowing, this primal encoding of potential, is accompanied by an equally innate and deeply embedded drive to manifest your implicit potential. It is a desire as potent as the hunger for your next meal. Entelechy is a spiritual instinct that pulls you forward like a full moon tide, back to the divine from which you came.

Entelechy is not something that can be proven by science. It cannot be analyzed, quantified, or predicted. We cannot dissect a leaf and discover its longing for the sun. For an alchemist, the belief in a person's innate drive to transform and become is partly a matter of careful observation and partly a matter of faith.

Problems, illness, and dysfunction arrive when the vital force of entelechy is blocked, ignored, or repressed. These problems may be physical, emotional, psychological, or spiritual, but they will show up somewhere in a person's life. Alchemical Healing teaches that blocks to entelechy are inevitable and necessary. They are a part of the experience of being in a body. These blocks refine you and serve as guideposts on the journey of your soul. The motion of entelechy is not linear. Rather, like the dance of life, it spirals and loops, stops, starts, and turns back on itself when it hits a hard place. Life is about flow, but also about resistance; it's through the resistance that you develop your spiritual muscles and learn the difficult work of turning lead to gold.

The Individuation Process

In Taoist alchemy, the innate drive to become the fullest possible expression of Who I Am is spoken of as the "return to Original Nature." The return to Origin is the goal of all Taoist alchemical practices. Through this return you come to know and accept who you are. You manifest your nature with the authenticity and spontaneity of a young child tempered by the illuminating wisdom of an elder. This is why one of the most revered Taoist philosophers and poets was given the honorific name Lao Tzu, which means old (or venerable) child. Paradoxically, *tzu* means both child and master. The Chinese understood that mastery comes when you can again be like a child, when after long years of practice and work you return to the pure spontaneous joy of your origins, the wholeness and perfection that were implicit in you at birth. This self-actualization is living one's Tao, living your life on Earth in accordance with the ways of Heaven.

From the viewpoint of Jungian archetypal psychology, the innate drive of the small self to become the fullest expression of the big Self is equally recognized as a human being's most important task, the central concern of a lifetime. Through the words you speak and the actions you take, you bring the finite and infinite more closely into alignment. Jung referred to this gradual realignment of self with Self as the process of individuation. Like the Taoists, Jung understood this process as a conscious return to a wholeness that we wordlessly remember, a knowing that infuses our being, our blood, and our bones. This wholeness—always just beyond our reach—beckons us closer to our own divinity.

As powerful and enlivening as our sexuality, our creativity, and our drives toward security and survival, this motivating impulse functions as a gyroscope constantly aligning and realigning us with our own True North. Illness, trauma, and suffering—whether physical, emotional, or spiritual—are in some way blocks or impasses on the journey but also opportunities to bring us back to a path we may have lost or to understand our path in some new and deeper way. Alchemical Healing is about getting a clearer sense of where you are going and removing impediments that interfere with getting there.

Putting It into Practice— Listening to the Heart

Alchemical Healing begins with the premise that every symptom is a signpost along the path of Tao and every treatment is an invitation to know the Self more deeply. However, when I began working with Margaret, it was difficult to see how her symptom could bring her closer to who she was truly meant to be.

Margaret reminded me of an Autumn morning after rain, when the hopeful sun peaks up over the horizon and edges each black tree branch with the barest sheen. She was frail and pale with only a hint of pink at the crest of her cheekbones. I saw her as a delicate silver lantern lit by a small and flickering flame.

Margaret was born with a dysfunctional heart valve and experienced troubling symptoms all her life. Heart palpitations, ongoing shortness of breath, weakness, dizziness, and sometimes fainting interfered with her ability to be active and socialize with her peers. While the possibility of replacing the valve had been discussed, her parents were wary of open-heart surgery and instead kept her home from school often and never allowed her to engage in the usual playground games, sports, and friendships of childhood.

She became a dreamer, a reader, and a loner. She lived with an ever-present sense of her own weakness and vulnerability. Because of her fear of breathlessness and fainting, she avoided going out or being with people she did not know well. Her isolation led to a profound lack of confidence and self-esteem. By the time we met, she was plagued by insomnia and disturbing dreams. She was ready to make changes in her life but did not know where to begin. Like her parents, she regarded surgery as a last resort and was hoping to find other ways to deal with her symptoms and care for her health. At twenty-five years old, she was still living at home with her parents, had no idea what she wanted to do with her life, and was very much debilitated by her heart condition.

With the agreement of her cardiologist, we began by working to alleviate some of the physical symptoms. The muscles of her chest and diaphragm had become constricted through long years of anxiety and inactivity and the qi in this area was blocked. I used needles to gently tonify the Heart and open flow between meridians. This made a big difference immediately; she was able to breathe more freely as the tightness in her chest diminished.

Although these first treatments helped somewhat with her physical symptoms, they did not shift her deep anxiety about her health and her reticence to move out into the world and live her life. I knew that if we were to effect change on this level, we would have to work on what I call the "spirit level." We would have to find a way to strengthen and stabilize the flickering flame in her lantern and strengthen the tenuous connection between her self and her Self.

I began by suggesting that she think of her body as a laboratory where she could be engaged in observation and learn about herself. There are no rights or wrongs in this laboratory, only information. As part of her lab work, I asked her to make note of when, why, and how her heart symptoms appeared, when they improved, and when they were exacerbated.

I chose to use very gentle techniques, such as flower essences, fine gauge needles, and simple meditation practices, as I did not want to further frighten or agitate her already traumatized shen with potent herbs, complex instructions, and overly forceful needle techniques. I asked her to make note of her dreams. I taught her a simple meditation developed by the HeartMath Institute to calm the heart and told her to practice it at least once a day.

Margaret's Simple Heart Meditation

Heart Focus: Begin by taking an easy inhalation and exhalation. Now, bring awareness to the place where you feel your heart, at the center of your chest or a bit over to the left side. You can place your hand over your heart to help you stay focused.

Heart Breathing: Pretend you are breathing through your heart area. Breathe slowly and gently (to a count of five or six) until your breathing feels smooth and balanced.

Heart Feeling: Continue to breathe through the area of your heart and identify a positive feeling, like appreciation for someone or something. You can recall a time when you felt unconditional love or care and re-experience that feeling now. It could be for a pet, a special place in nature, or an activity that was fun. Once you have found a positive feeling, sustain this feeling by continuing heart focus, heart breathing, and heart feeling.

I taught Margaret a technique called "Moving It Over" drawn from Focusing, which is a simple yet powerful body awareness process developed by philosopher Eugene Gendlin. I explained to Margaret, paraphrasing one my favorite Gendlin lines, that you can't tell what the soup tastes like when you stick your whole head in the pot. In other words, when you create a little distance, a comfortable space between you, your symptom, and all the associated emotional drama, you can actually come into relationship to the feelings and understand the messages they want you to hear. For some people, it's easy right away and for others it takes a lot of practice, but if you stay with it, Moving It Over often has surprisingly gratifying results.

Moving It Over Practice

- Begin by bringing awareness to the body. Feel your feet on the floor, back against the chair, your breath going in and out of your chest.

- Then, invite your awareness to gather at the place where you feel the physical symptom or the effect of the troubling emotion.

- Explore what you feel inside your inner laboratory. Take some time to bring it into focus. The feeling may be vague or clear and it may change as you pay attention to it. In Focusing, the feeling you find when you shine your awareness inside is called a "Body Felt Sense."

- Without judgment or trying to change anything, just say hello to what you find. See if you can find a word or an image that describes it.

- Now, imagine you could gather up the Body Felt Sense and move it just a little bit away from the center of you. Play with distance. Maybe it feels good to let it be where it is or just a bit out of your body for a moment. Or maybe you want to move it far away for the rest of the day. And sometimes, with some really difficult feelings, you want to wrap them up and send them down a river and out to the sea forever. You are free to imagine whatever you like in this exercise as long as it feels like something moves inside of you. You are looking to feel more relaxed, to have more room inside, to hear your inner voice more clearly.

The ultimate goal of Moving It Over is to make more space for the Self to get through to you!

Last but definitely not least, I recommended that Margaret take the flower essence Mimulus. Mimulus is a low-growing shrub with small flowers shaped like monkey faces or tiny lustrous colored masks. The name *Mimulus* comes from the Latin *mimus*, which means "mime" or "actor," one who wears a mask. When made into a flower essence, Mimulus is a remedy for known fears. It is the flower to call on when we are frightened or anxious about something real, something that we can name and describe, even if it has not yet happened; for example, Margaret's fear of fainting. In addition, Mimulus is recommended when there is great, even excessive, sensitivity and fragility, when the timidity that naturally arises with concerns about something immediate and real becomes a generalized, persistent, and tormenting anxiety. The Mimulus person lives behind a mask of fear.

Margaret was dedicated to her healing process. Although she was not immediately aware of any marked change, with careful self-observation she began to recognize that her symptoms of heart palpitations and chest tightness usually coincided with an emotional upset. Sometimes it was her own emotion, but more frequently it was when she felt someone else's upset. What was even more striking was that the worst symptoms came when she was in the presence of someone who was trying to hide feelings from Margaret or from themselves. She realized that even when the person wasn't aware that they were having an emotion or an upset, she could clearly feel the emotion. Her heart would tell her in no uncertain terms that something was up. This discovery was new and interesting information, but we had yet to see any dramatic change in how she was feeling. Her reticence, shyness, anxiety, and lack of self-esteem were all still present.

Then one day she came in looking radiant. Her whole demeanor had changed. She told me she was reading a book and came across the phrase, "What we consider our greatest weakness is often our greatest gift." At that moment, something shifted for Margaret.

I will never forget when the aha moments started happening, when the pieces started coming together for me in a sort of wild internal dance that literally had me gripping the sides of my chair. It is only while I sat there, absorbing these words, that I realized how wrong I had been all these years, how my heart valve was not faulty at all—how it was, in fact, a most powerful healing tool that allowed me to feel, at a very deep level, not only my own emotions, but also the emotions of others.

Margaret opened to an encounter with her Self. In her own words, the encounter disrupted her ordinary state of being, broke through her habitual thought patterns, and left her "literally gripping the sides of her chair." With time and patience, our work had culminated in a breakthrough, a fundamental shift in Margaret's sense of who she was and who she could become. Through this encounter with the Self, she recognized that she was much bigger than her symptoms, bigger than the fragile person she had known herself to be. She realized that what she had viewed as a lifelong weakness could also be a strength. Through the recognition of her acute sensitivity to other people's feelings and emotions, Margaret at last understood that her illness had given her a gift.

Not long after that session, Margaret decided to apply to a graduate program in marriage and family therapy. After being accepted, she moved out of her parents' home and into an apartment with other students. She now works as a counselor and listens to the guidance of her heart daily.

Chapter 5

Inner Work = Outer Change

Change is coming—what do we have to imagine as we prepare for it?
—Adrienne Maree Brown, *Emergent Strategy*

Reversing the Light

In 1997, I attended a workshop on ecopsychology, grief, and environmental despair led by Buddhist scholar and environmental activist Joanna Macy. That weekend affirmed a hunch I had about personal and planetary change. I became more convinced than ever that the healing we do inside, at the level of attitude, presence, and inner response patterns, has an effect on the quality and impact of our actions in the outer world.

Macy identified a "shift in human consciousness" as the single most important factor in preserving our natural resources and restoring health to our ecosystems. She affirmed the necessity for engaged political action but said that a change in our collective attitude toward our emotional and physical bodies, a restoration of empathy with other living creatures, and a renewal of the ancient understanding that all matter is sacred could ultimately alter the reality human beings create on the ground. For Macy, the inner work of shifting the way we organize our experience of the world is crucial, even primary, to the healing of our planet. In order to realize this shift, people have to come out of denial and disassociation from their own bodies and emotions and feel their grief in response to species extinction, the destruction of forests, and the loss of connection to the divine wisdom of nature. My takeaway was that healing begins when we realize our unity with the world and the intrinsic connection between inner and outer reality.

In the many years that have passed since that weekend retreat, I have worked with hundreds of patients, students, and other fellow travelers. As a practitioner, teacher, supervisor, mother, partner, writer, and artist, I practice and facilitate processes of healing/wholing and change in my own and other people's lives. If there is one trend that emerges, it is that most of the lasting and positive change I see in people's outer lives begins with an internal shift. I repeatedly see this seemingly inexplicable synergy or reciprocity play out in my patients' lives. For example, the African American woman who finally got her first solo exhibition after coming to terms with her ancestral slave trauma and the fear of ambition that she carried in her own body; the reclusive carpenter who, after two decades of living alone in an isolated trailer in the woods, met a woman and fell in love after finding the courage to face the violence he experienced during his early home life; the depressed alcoholic who stopped blaming her husband for her unhappiness and found joy once she got sober and became a vocal activist for immigration reform.

The outer effects of our actions depend on the inner state of our hearts and souls. Although there are tangible conditions—oppression, poverty, and illness—that prevent human beings from actualizing the potential of the Self, I believe that the greatest impediment of all is the inability to look within and engage some form of inner spiritual work.

In alchemical language, when I see transformation that actually changes the shape, direction, and outcome of a person's life, the process is driven by conscious alignment with entelechy. I witness an awakening that quickens the soul forces and drives what is implicit, ideal, and imaginable toward the manifest and real. In other words, the outer forms of life blossom from an inner seed. It is our recognition, care, and cultivation of the seed that determines the quality and expression of its blossom.

The Alchemy of Inner Work

Inner Work

The original alchemical texts were intentionally written in obscure language to make sure the powerful practices they described did not fall into the hands of the "wrong people" who would misuse them to further their outer ambitions rather than their inner spiritual development. The obscurity of the language was meant to protect the secrets but also to provide a psychic labyrinth of symbols, riddles, and poetry that engages the reader with the text in a slow, gradual, and embodied way that is, in itself, a spiritual practice. When I first came across the idea of "turning the light" in one of my favorite Taoist alchemical texts, *The Secret of the Golden Flower*, or what in other texts is referred to as "reversing the handle of the stars," I was intrigued but confused. Initially, I skimmed over the phrase mistaking it for an antiquated meaningless reference; however, seeing the idea repeated in a variety of ways in multiple texts, I grew determined to decode the message.

After many years of meditation, I came to understand that this phrase contains in shorthand form an essential clue to understanding the alchemical project. The light referred to in the Taoist texts is the evanescent gleam of the "true gold." It is the igniting fire of spirit that sparks like starlight in the eyes of a healthy human being, the illumination of self-awareness that waits for discovery, hidden deep in the heart of matter.

For alchemists, this consciousness or spirit within matter is not an invisible abstraction but an emanation of the divine that we can perceive when our hearts are open and receptive. Every human being is born with this light. You see it looking back at you from the eyes of an infant or from the loving gaze of a friend. This light has the power to awaken conscious awareness. Yet the tremendous spiritual potency of this light seed remains dormant until a person makes the critical decision to cultivate it.

The Taoist texts emphasize that, "This light is easily stirred and hard to stabilize." Without the engagement of a stabilizing conscious will, the yang light of the shen shines outward, captivated by the glamor of matter, consuming its potency in a frenzy of extroverted activity, draining psychic energy in an entropic spin of desire and disappointment, loves and losses, attachment and reactivity. Propaganda, advertising, gaming, and the entire entertainment industry capitalizes on this tendency for the yang nature of consciousness to be ensnared by outer impressions. It takes a great deal of effort to reverse its direction and pay attention to the world within, but this single mindful action is at the root of all alchemical practice.

The great insight of the early alchemists was that every person is born with the capacity to intentionally cultivate this star seed of light. But this capacity, while intrinsic to human nature and, as you will see, to human neurobiology, does not function involuntarily. It requires a counterintuitive flipping of a switch, a willful engagement that shifts attention from the outer to the inner world, a readiness to focus not on your thoughts but on the source of the mind, particularly on the "open center"—the spacious awareness of the heart. This practice is the backward spin, the *contra natura*—the conscious decision to interrupt a natural flow in service of spiritual growth and deeper understanding—that alchemists recognized as the first step in alchemy.

However, as modern-day alchemist and poet Jay Ramsay reminds us, "Alchemy takes time like love takes time." It is not enough to turn the light around once. Alchemical healing and the accompanying expansion of awareness requires work and there is no pill you can take that will do the work for you. Unlike the immediate awakening of spiritual revelation or the induced brain chemistry changes due to hallucinogenic influence or pharmaceutical intervention, the embodied soul-level changes and reorganization of neural circuitry of inner alchemy do not just happen to you. They arise from conscious, devoted practice over time. Engaging your will to interrupt the automatic extroverted gaze and bring focus back to your interior, not once but again and again in a yin, slow process of ongoing cultivation gradually roots and stabilizes the yang shen, so that the star seed naturally flowers in its own right time.

The ultimate goal of this gradual, patient inner work is self-awareness. This spacious self-awareness includes not only your conscious ego and physical body but also your psychic experiences, dreams, feelings, fantasies, and bodily animal knowing. It is what allows you to transform your inner lead—your stuck behavior patterns, resentments, envy, and other negative emotions and unconscious reactivities—into wisdom, compassion, authentic spontaneity, and effective responsiveness to the outer environment. It is what connects you to your big Self and brings your daily life closer to your Tao. *The Secret of the Golden Flower* states it simply: "Once you turn the light around, everything in the world is also turned around."

You Are Wired for Self-Awareness

Some time after I deciphered the meaning of reversing the light and recognized its centrality to alchemy, I discovered the research of physician and trauma specialist Bessel van der Kolk. His book *The Body Keeps the Score*, along with other recent discoveries in neurobiology, confirmed my hunches. The research also affirmed for me the significance of the alchemical practices related to "light reversal," not only for my own personal inner work and my clinical work with patients but also for humanity as a whole.

In the early 1990s, medical researchers developed new technology that allows them to look inside the brain to see what occurs when a person is feeling a particular emotion or thinking about a specific idea. By combining positron emission tomography (PET scans) with functional magnetic resonance imaging (fMRI), scientists were able for the first time to observe the functioning brain in real time and to map the circuitry of consciousness.

Through rigorously controlled experiments and careful research, neuroscientists discovered that the part of the nervous system that regulates emotions and instinctual reactions to stress and trauma is lodged deep in ancient sectors of the brain: the limbic system and brainstem. Imagine you have a powerful wild animal living in the center of your nervous system that believes its sole job is to maintain your survival at whatever cost. Or there is an old malfunctioning Fire Alarm in your head that goes off randomly at the slightest whiff of smoke, whether the source is a bit of burned toast or the house burning down, with no capacity to discern the source of actual danger. Sound familiar? That's because it's how this part of your brain reacts to real or perceived danger and stress, particularly if you've experienced any kind of trauma or if you live in the unpredictable chaos of the modern world!

There is another part of your brain that is in charge of what psychologists call the "executive function." Your capacity for planning, critical thought, and logic is located in the neocortex, evolutionarily the most recently formed frontal lobes of your brain. This aspect of the nervous system, which van der Kolk refers to as the Watchtower, allows us to hover calmly over our thoughts, emotions, and bodily sensations while we rationally appraise a situation, assess the validity of our instinctual responses (that is, determine whether the smoke is coming from the toaster or from the house burning down), and then to strategize appropriate and effective responses to events around us. A well-functioning Watchtower modulates the Fire Alarm and helps you remain in conscious relationship to yourself, to others, and to your Tao.

However, as proven by real-time neuro-imaging, when you are under stress or experiencing strong emotions, the connection between the frontal lobes and the more primitive parts of your brain shuts down. The Fire Alarm danger detector overrides the Watchtower executive function. The alarm gets so loud it disrupts any rational capacity to accurately perceive the reality of threat or organize sensory data into a coherent story.

As a result of the interruption of these lines of communication, our instinctual survival drives remain mostly unconscious and unevaluated by our critical mind. The primal instincts of the animal take control and the part of us that could care for, love, temper, and channel that vital wildness is overshadowed. Under these conditions, human beings react to the world in survival-driven, irrational, and inflammatory ways that create ongoing cycles of suffering. When this happens, it becomes virtually impossible to hear the messages of the Self or to perceive the path of your Tao because the focus of your attention is oriented outward.

And yet, just as the ancient Taoist alchemists recognized that human beings are born with an innate capacity to interrupt the entropic yang activity of the shen, modern scientists now recognize that we are born with an innate capacity to restore communication between the disparate parts of our brain, between the Fire Alarm and the Watchtower, the Wild Animal of the limbic system/brain stem and the Caring Friend of the higher mind. The amazing truth is that you are born already wired with the ability to consciously contact, nurture, and transform the reactive wild animal of your instinctual body into a responsive helpful ally and a trustworthy guide.

While most of your conscious brain is focused on the outside world, on analyzing data and planning strategic responses, there is a special part of the frontal lobes called the "medial prefrontal cortex" (MPFC), located directly above and behind your eyes at the point Vedic alchemists called the "third eye." This special and very recently developed part of your brain notices what is going on inside of you and allows you to consciously recognize, evaluate, and care about what you are feeling. The primary function of the MPFC can best be described as self-awareness; it is the only reliable conduit of communication between your conscious mind, your emotions, and the instinctual wisdom of your body.

Psychologists, brain researchers, and trauma specialists have been studying the MPFC and its effect on the emotional body for the past three decades. There is no doubt that the MPFC endows us with the ability to modulate our emotions, to recognize what is going on inside of us, and to consciously communicate with the deep wisdom of our animal body. But the MPFC does not function involuntarily, especially when we are traumatized, under stress, or emotionally activated. Modern research parallels the insights of the ancient alchemists: the alteration of our emotions, our instinctual reactivity, and our patterns of habitual behavior begin with a reversal of awareness, a counter-intuitive flipping of the neurological switch, a turning around of the inner eye. Change in your life begins when you shift the focus of your attention away from the outer world—the others who are wronging you and the events you cannot control— and instead drop down from your thinking mind into the deep yin spaciousness of your heart.

The enormous psycho-spiritual importance of this connection was recognized by ancient alchemists and is depicted in the Tarot, a deck of seventy-eight cards used from the mid-fifteenth century throughout Europe. The Tarot offers a symbolic map of consciousness that has the potential to guide the seeker through a journey of spiritual growth. The Eleventh Major Arcana Card: Strength (in some decks numbered Eight) depicts a beautiful woman gently taming and guiding the lion by her side. The strength this card portrays is not a dominating power of one being over another but rather a harmonious relationship between two aspects of being—the instinctual animal body symbolized by the lion and the refining spirit of the mind represented by the serene woman with her hand resting lovingly on the lion's head. Here, the woman's gaze is not focused on the outer world but is turned inward and down toward the animal who looks back at her with devoted adoration. The card can be understood as a picture of Sophia, the Goddess of Wisdom, tempering the primitive fiery yang energy of the wild beast. The infinity sign that floats like a crown or halo above the woman's head symbolizes the ongoing renewal of the life force when these opposing forces come into the right relationship.

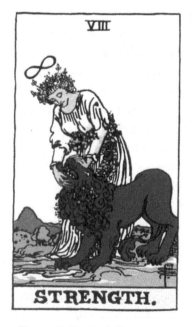

Figure 8. Strength Tarot card

The Alchemy of Inner Work

Practicing the Pause

Most spiritual traditions, including alchemy, understand that the human tendency to act out—to react to a situation impulsively or emotionally from instinctual survival drives without the mediation of the conscious mind—is a major cause of suffering. From a modern scientific point of view, the Pause is the first step taken to interrupt this reactivity, reorganizing the circuitry of your nervous system and shifting entrenched neurological patterns. From an alchemical perspective, it is the first step in reversing the light—sometimes referred to as "stopping"—and it is the catalytic agent of inner alchemy. By using the will to momentarily interrupt an instinctually driven habitual or reactive behavior, you re-establish the right relationship between your MPFC and your limbic system.

In bringing the compassionate hand of your will to calm and quiet the wild animal of your limbic system and brain stem, you create a space between the external stimulus and your gut-level reaction, and you make room for a new possibility to come to life. The *Secret of the Golden Flower* reminds us, "A breath-pause means a year according to human time and a hundred years measured by the long night of reincarnation." In the space of a moment, the infinite rests.

The insight or response that arises from this stillness will be something you could not have figured out with your conscious mind or activated through your instincts. Instead, the information will come from your body and you can trust that it will bring you closer to your Tao.

Practicing the Pause

Recognize that you are in a situation where you would ordinarily react habitually, instinctually, or emotionally.

Stop!

Feel the hand of your will calming down your inner animal.

Invite your awareness away from the outer situation to the space around your heart.

Take three long, slow breaths.

Notice what happens.

If, after the Pause, you still feel the drive to react impulsively, hold on to the reins of your animal a bit longer and repeat the mantra:

Pause . . . Breathe . . . Remember . . .

The Pause creates a space in which you can re-equilibrate and reorient to your higher Self. The I Ching tells us in Hexagram 52—Keeping Still, Mountain,

> True quiet means keeping still when the time has come to keep still and going forward when the time has come to go forward. In this way rest and movement are in agreement with the demands of the time, and there is a light in life . . . when a person has thus become calm, he may turn to the outside world . . . whoever acts from these deep levels makes no mistakes.

Inner and Outer Alchemy

Alchemy has two faces. One looks out at manifest form: the elements, ores, minerals, plants, and animals of the natural world. The other looks in at imaginal form: the dreams, fantasies, and *archetypes* of the psyche. One involves work in the outer laboratory of matter and the other in the inner laboratory of the soul. In China, these two gazes were related to *waidan*, outer alchemy that focused on compounding and transforming natural substances, and *neidan*, inner alchemy that focused on transforming internal spiritual essences. Yet, inner alchemists employ the language of outer alchemy to describe their practices and experiences and outer traditions depend on the expanded sight of inner alchemy to access the mysteries of matter.

The alchemical viewpoint is that inner and outer worlds intermingle and are mutually influential. Just as modern quantum physicists are discovering that the observer affects the observed, alchemists understood that the eye that perceives also affects what is being perceived. The matter we work with also works with us. To the outer alchemist, the mercury, mandrake root, or St. John's Wort is not just a bit of inert matter waiting passively to be worked on but rather a living, sentient bit of psyche with its own wisdom and intentionality. To the inner alchemist, the dream image that comes with a message at midnight still lives at her side as a living, breathing entity the next day. The dream image, the mandrake root, and the mercury are present with their own impulses and personalities, subjects of their own story, each unique and capable of relationship. In the alchemical laboratory, it is understood that matter responds to our psychic and emotional states, and the spiritual awakening of the alchemist is intrinsically connected to the transformation of the matter being worked on. Inner and outer processes of change are interdependent.

Despite the division of alchemy into two separate lines of investigation, there is only one alchemy. This unified art combines the inner and outer gaze into an expanded awareness that penetrates beyond the outer edges of form to touch the ephemeral spirit that is embedded in matter. As we immerse ourselves in this wisdom of the past, we discover a portal through which we can enter the new, nonlinear, multi-dimensional integral world of the future.

The Irruption of Integrality

Along with Macy's emphasis on the central importance of consciousness and van der Kolk's insights regarding the destructive effects of trauma on the nervous system, Jean Gebser's seminal book *The Ever-Present Origin* has had a profound influence on the development of my ideas about healing.

Born in Posen, Germany, in 1905, Gebser was a philosopher, linguist, poet, and spiritual visionary. As a student in Munich, he witnessed firsthand the sadistic violence of the *Sturmabteilung*, or Storm Detachment, the hordes of Nazi Brownshirts who roamed through the city streets of Germany beginning in the 1920s. Horrified by what he recognized as the rise of fascism in his homeland, Gebser fled to Spain. Soon after, with the outbreak of the Spanish Civil War, he fled to Paris, before finally finding safety in Switzerland.

During his university years, Gebser was inspired by his readings of Rainer Maria Rilke, Sigmund Freud, C. G. Jung, and Arthur Schopenhauer. But it was later, in Madrid and Paris, that his true intellectual and spiritual awakening was catalyzed by personal encounters with Pablo Neruda, Pablo Picasso, André Malraux, and the circle of artists and writers that gathered around them. In the midst of the danger and chaos in Europe preceding the Second World War, Gebser found himself at the epicenter of the prophetic creativity of modernism. He could clearly see that the world he had known as a child in Germany was disintegrating. At the same time, he recognized the stirrings of something vital and new.

As Europe headed inexorably toward war, the vast array of new ideas and art forms Gebser encountered came together in a flash of insight, a vision of the evolution of human consciousness that would inspire and sustain him for the rest of his life. Despite the turmoil, death, and destruction of his time, he became convinced that something vigorously creative was simultaneously coming to life. Rather than foreshadowing an inevitable disaster, he came to believe that the crisis of modern culture was actually the beginning of a vital restructuring. In the midst of the breakdown of familiar, old beliefs and cultural assumptions, he perceived a new consciousness emerging from the ashes of the old. With Einstein's discovery of relativity in science, the development of cubism and surrealism in painting, Freud's exploration of the unconscious in psychology, and the upsurge of Western interest in mysticism, Eastern religions, and healing methods, the fixed divisions central to Cartesian rationalism were beginning to dissolve.

Gebser's project, which occupied him for the rest of his life until he died in 1972, was to demonstrate the evolution of consciousness by exploring the artistic, philosophical, and spiritual expressions of human beings over time. Through the intensive study of prehistoric cave art; Aztec poetry; Anatolian, Greek, and Roman mythology; sculpture and architecture; medieval and renaissance painting; as well as the art, psychology, and science of the twentieth century, Gebser was able to delineate distinct worldviews that he referred to as "structures of consciousness."

Gebser identified three main worldviews that underlie our own mental consciousness—the name Gebser assigned to the dualistic, linear, rationally oriented way we currently view the world. He

The Alchemy of Inner Work

named the earlier structures archaic (pre-historic), magical (Neolithic tribal/hunter gatherer/tool-making), and mythical (early settlement/agricultural/myth-making). Most importantly, he went on to say that these "earlier" structures of consciousness are "ever-present." Although relatively dormant, they still exist in us right now.

The evolution of these structures of consciousness that has taken place over the course of millennia happens on an individual level throughout a lifetime. As a fetus, you bathed in the timeless, spaceless ocean of the archaic as you swam in the embryonic waters of your mother's womb. You return to this archaic state each night when you drift into the unconsciousness of deep sleep, open to the ego-less states of certain forms of meditation, or experience the brief but profoundly restorative rest of Shavasana at the closing of a yoga class. The shamanic magician came to life when, as an infant, you grasped a spoon and began tapping rhythms on a table, exultating in the powerful new ability to send vibration through space. You become a magician again when you dance to the driving beat of drums, communicate nonverbally with your pet, telepathically know that your brother is about to call before the phone rings, or know "in your bones" not to walk down a particular alley at twilight. You discovered the mythical with the first fairy tale that enthralled you, the first story you told about an imaginary friend. Mythical consciousness returns each time you are moved by a great movie, fascinated by a royal wedding, or touched by the mysterious symbols of a dream.

By observing changes in art, architecture, and other cultural expressions in relationship to the chronology of historical events, Gebser also noted that old structures devolved into inefficiency and new, more efficient ones emerged at pivotal moments in human history. These pivot points occur when an old way of being or predominant worldview was no longer capable of offering solutions to the challenges facing human beings at a given time. For example, the free-ranging hunter-gatherers of the magical era followed the wild herds and foraging trails in their ceaseless wanderings until they were forced by the growing human population and declining wild animal populations to settle down and discover new ways to nourish themselves. This led to the cultivation of fruits and vegetables and the domestication of farm animals, which in turn necessitated the prediction of seasonal patterns and the development of calendars. In this way, magical consciousness was eclipsed by the mythical. The drumming, chanting, telepathically transmitted traditions of shamanism were overshadowed by the laboratory observations and written documentations of alchemy. Very real environmental challenges catalyzed the emergence of neurological, logical, and spiritual capacities that were already present yet, until then, dormant in human beings. At the same time, the outer world was drastically changed as agriculture, technology, and longer-living human populations altered the very shape, texture, and atmosphere of the natural environment.

Like Gebser, I believe we are now living at another pivotal moment of new consciousness irruption. Like the hunter-gathering people who evolved to discover agriculture, astronomy, writing, and metallurgy in order to survive, we are compelled by the conditions of our time to discover new forms of awareness, new tools, and new skills that will allow not only ourselves but also our planet to survive. The cause-effect logic and adherence to radical divisive dichotomies of our current mental structure are useless in the face of the complex, multi-dimensional challenges of the twenty-first century. Every day, I see the deteriorating efficiency of this separating attitude in the intractable conflicts within our two-party political system, the persistent animosity between people of different races and religions, the prophetic rejection by many people of the notion of defined binary gender, the alienation of my patients from nature and their own bodies, and the absurd and pointless divisive arguments on Facebook comment threads.

In order to grapple with the infinite array of vectors—both physical and psychological—that have converged to result in climate change, the decimation of the environment, immigrant crises and refugee caravans, new strains of resistant pathogens, immune dysfunction, rampant addiction, and the impasses of our health care systems, we need to find new ways of perceiving and understanding data. We must cultivate new attitudes toward life and death, self and other, as well as to our environment. We need to literally learn to see the world differently.

The Alchemy of Inner Work

Mental consciousness, which began with the discovery of individual perspective during the Italian Renaissance and the advent of modern science and medicine in Europe in the 1600s, is being eclipsed by a new structure that Gebser called the "integral." Integrality, whose first whispers began at the turn of the twentieth century, emerged alongside the budding awareness that time is relative rather than linear and the understanding that past, present, and future exist simultaneously not only in the universe, but also in us. Integrality will continue to emerge as we become consciously aware that the earlier forms of consciousness still exist in us as unconscious yet highly active influences. By rendering time transparent, we perceive not only through our current mental consciousness but also through the archaic, magical, and mythical ways that humans have always understood the world. Integrality emerges as we bring these various forms of consciousness into awareness simultaneously.

Integrality constellates in us as we surrender the primacy of our materialistic, outer-directed, mental viewpoint and honor all our various ways of knowing. It happens, for example, when instead of just treating opioid addiction by developing pharmaceutical drugs that reduce cravings, we also address the underlying factors that influence how people feel—the alienation from place, community, and self and the accompanying loss of spirit that leads to addiction as well as anxiety, depression, and suicide. It happens when instead of endlessly arguing about how to cover the sky-rocketing cost of pharmaceuticals, high-tech surgeries, and long-term care for an increasingly aging population, we allow ourselves to feel the pain of human suffering and take time to re-evaluate the assumptions and values underlying our attitudes toward health.

Integrality demands that we sacrifice the you/me, good/bad, right/wrong point of view and linear cause and effect logic that dominates our culture. It begins with the willingness to not know, to be curious about a perspective other than your own. With the irruption of integrality, we are called to bear the discomfort and disorientation of opening to the other less familiar structures of consciousness. As we begin to access and care about the intelligence of the natural world, the wisdom of our bodies, the diversity of our respective inner feelings, and our irrational intuitions and mysterious dreams, we may also begin to discover surprising solutions to seemingly insoluble problems.

Pause. Wait. Listen to the small, new voice that leads you away from outer blame to inner responsibility, away from addictive behavior toward self-care, away from compulsive acting out toward inner contemplation. Trust that these small but massively difficult inner shifts will begin to have an effect on the world around you.

We are all longing, whether we know it or not, for a more efficient and more spacious way of being human. Yet the path is not straightforward. From a cursory look at breakthrough moments in human history such as Copernicus's realization that the Earth circled the sun rather than vice versa, Darwin's theory of evolution, the civil rights movement, or even the body/mind medicine of our time, we see that the innovation, creativity, and excitement of the new is always accompanied by a tendency in some to cling to the inefficient but familiar past rather than take the risk of diving into an unknown future.

These regressive tendencies show up as rigid fundamentalism in politics and religion and an ever-growing dependency on paternalistic authorities who promise one-sided solutions and simple quick fixes, whether through fascist dictatorships, corporate advertising, or prohibitively costly pharmaceutical interventions. When you are stressed, confused, or sick, the limbic-driven survival tendency to grasp for the regressive safety of unconscious responses is especially strong. You instinctively reach for the magic pill when you are in pain and pray for the shamanic powers of your practitioner to offer the fix when something goes wrong with your body.

For me, the treatment room has been my laboratory, the safe space where I explore the dance of these various structures of consciousness with my patients and watch for the astonishing irruptions of integrality. I begin at the mental level with a carefully recorded, linear health history that gives me the "facts of the matter" and identifies a patient's presenting issue. I then move into the mythical as I listen with my emotional body to the feeling tone of a person's story

The Alchemy of Inner Work

and tease out the larger life themes at play. The magical comes alive in the nonverbal cues we exchange, the body language and rhythms that underlie our verbal conversation. The moment a patient lies down on the treatment table and I take the pulses, our breathing changes, words disappear into silence, and the archaic comes back from dormancy. And it is then, when all these structures unfold one upon the other like the petals of a transparent flower, that something I cannot ever fully explain occurs. Now is when Michaela's coyotes arrive and both she and I see them. Now is when I instinctually know that it is time to call on a particular flower essence, touch a particular point with a specific essential oil, or walk around that fourth side of the dark pond to face the unknown.

As we move into integral awareness, we become like the master practitioners of old whose gaze penetrated into the invisible spaces between the surfaces of things, who saw the world through the eyes of an open and attentive heart. When we recognize that the material world is illuminated and animated by the immaterial, that time and space are holographic rather than linear phenomenon, and that our own flesh is inspired with a heavenly breath, then in the words of the Chinese medical text *The Yellow Emperor's Classic of Internal Medicine*, spirit becomes clear to us "[a]s though the wind has blown away the clouds." Through this penetrating illumination, something new comes to life, a way of looking at the healing process that frees us from the limits of dualistic thinking, the terror of death as an enemy, the devitalizing grip of materialism, and the isolation of linear time and space-bound existence. For me, the primary goal of healing at the present time should be supporting human beings in moving through the fear, confusion, and doubt that are an inevitable and necessary part of reorganization at this fundamental level of our being.

Gebser's vision helped me articulate what I perceive as the first intimations of an emerging, more life-sustaining and efficient consciousness. It also helped me understand why going back to retrieve the wisdom of the past is a necessary step in this emergence. On the days when the stories of violence, greed, and suffering become too much for me to bear, Gebser's carefully researched, sweeping yet elegantly structured vision gives me hope that despite all appearances to the contrary, human consciousness is up to something and it is worth getting up in the morning to participate in the effort.

Alchemists live in a world of interconnected beings that include humans, animals, plants, metals, minerals, microbes, and a vast community of nonphysical spirit entities whose intelligence interfaces with our own. As an alchemist, I can see from my own point of view but also from the perspective of the rivers and waterways, the trees and forests, the sunlight and open fields, the stones and the mountains, and the wild ones who speak to me in my dreams.

Alchemical Healing's emphasis on the inner life does not eliminate the need for concerted and courageous acts of service and healing in the outer world. In contrast to the human potential and New Age movements of the past four decades that focused on personal growth and individual experience, Alchemical Healing echoes the wisdom of ancient times when it was understood that the well-being of humans and the world are interdependent. It aligns with current social justice movements that insist on the centrality of fair and just relations between individuals and the larger society as well as with all beings on the planet we share. And now, as alchemy moves from the past into the future, it collides with recent findings of quantum physics that demonstrate the interconnectedness of matter and consciousness. I am convinced that outer work without inner healing is unsustainable and will not succeed, and inner work that does not find an outlet to the larger world is ultimately something of a dead end.

It is time to bring the hidden esoteric concepts and practices of alchemy out from hiding. Unless we can integrate the various structures within our consciousness, befriend the Wild Animal that lives within our nervous systems, and learn to value the gifts of our inner world, it is unlikely that we will survive as a species for much longer.

The radical leap presented in this book is that our inner and outer worlds are not separate but exist on a continuum of connection and communication. The slow, difficult shifts we make inside as we take responsibility for our own thoughts, emotions, and actions are mirrored in our outer experiences. Although we recognize that the challenges currently facing humanity on environmental, economic, and political levels seem insurmountable, we still believe that some level of healing is always possible and that it begins with a shift in consciousness, with inner work that leads to outer change. In Part Two, you will learn practices and tools, and be introduced to medicinal substances that will help you bring this integral reality and new way of healing into your life.

Part Two

Entering the Laboratory

Chapter 6

The Keys to Your Laboratory

Alchemy begins before we enter the mine, the forge, or laboratory. It begins in the blue vault, the seas, in the mind's thinking in images, imagining ideationally, speculatively, in words that are both images and ideas, in words that turn things into flashing ideas and ideas into little things that crawl, the blue power of the word itself.

—James Hillman, *A Blue Fire*

The Laboratory

You begin the work of alchemy by stepping into a laboratory—a protected place where you do intentional, conscious creative work. The laboratory might be a treatment room where you heal, a journal where you write, a studio where you paint, a garden where you cultivate vegetables, or a designated space where you meditate or read. It could be your kitchen, your bedroom, your body, or a tent in the wilderness. It could be a friendship, a group, a marriage, or an ongoing, therapeutic relationship.

The matter is the medium you are exploring. It can be pigment, soil, soup, anger, grief, love, your vision for the future, or the wounds of childhood still haunting your current life. It can be a dream. It is always connected to your soul.

The tools are the things you find in your hand and hold in your heart.

From an alchemical perspective, your laboratory is a sacred space where something new gestates and comes to life. It must have certain womb-like qualities, including protection, defined limits, seclusion, and the capacity to remain intact until a process is complete.

The laboratory can be any place in the world you inhabit. What distinguishes it from other ordinary places is the key you use to enter. Ideally, the whole of your life will become a living laboratory.

In this chapter, I share keys that have opened the door to my own laboratory again and again. I turn to these keys when I need to understand my physical symptoms, my emotional upsets, and my dreams. I rely on them when I face big decisions. Daily, these keys help me stay on track and aligned with what is best for me, from deciding whether to say yes or no to an invitation, to knowing what foods I need to eat to nourish my body, to adjusting my work schedule when I'm feeling pushed to my edges. I bring these keys with me every time I walk into the treatment room. I teach them to my patients who use them to make medical decisions—whether or not to take anti-depressants or to follow the doctor's recommendation of chemotherapy after surgery—as well as personal and professional life choices. These keys are the touchstones that can help you keep your focus and faith in the midst of the destabilizing uncertainties, moral challenges, and chaos of our changing world.

Find the Truth from Within Your Own Being

The foundational Emerald Tablet of European alchemy was carved on a block of liquid emerald that later crystallized to gemstone. As the story goes, it was discovered in a cave by Alexander the Great when he conquered Egypt in 332 BCE, but its actual origins remain unknown. The first precept or key of the Emerald Tablet sets the tone for all alchemical work: search relentlessly for truth.

From the start, alchemy has been about the discovery of the secret truth of life itself. Alchemists understood that the exploration begins right here in the present moment, in the place where your feet stand. Search from within. Trust your own knowing. Listen to your senses and your heart.

Alchemy is an independent and unconventional tradition that champions personal vision, experimentation, idiosyncratic practices, and unorthodox spirituality. Alchemists think for themselves. This truth explains why the secret art has always posed a threat to organized religion, authoritarian leadership, and fundamentalist attitudes whose validity and power depend on the acceptance of an enforced, one-size-fits all reality.

The First Key

Begin by doubting everything you think you know. Sacrifice certainty. Get curious.

Leave behind your habitual way of being and enter the world as if it were a dream. Ask yourself: Why did this weed decide to grow beside my front door? Why are so many angry people crossing my path this week? What is it about this corner of the garden that makes me feel so happy?

Look at the world anew. See the sky as an ocean. Imagine trees with their branches as roots reaching down to the stars. Cherish your challenging friends as teachers and your troubles as possibilities for growth.

As Above, So Below

Ancient Taoist alchemists viewed nature as the "visible face of Tao." The world you see reflects an unseen world that shimmers just beyond the veil of form. The configurations of the constellations in the infinite sky above are mirrored in the patterns of your daily life on Earth below.

From an alchemical perspective, Heaven and Earth, Above and Below, are equal partners in the dance of life. But when it came to distilling a drop of the One Thing—the agent of transformation—alchemists looked downward. Alchemy invites you to recognize that matter, including your body and all the organic forms of life on Earth, is not just inert "stuff" to be weighed and manipulated, analyzed and fixed, commodified and used, but holds energetic patterns and crystallized vibrations that express active, divine intelligence. The more you bring your soul's gaze to the material world, the more it will come alive to you. In alchemy, as in a dream, anything can be your teacher.

The Second Key

All you need to begin is a stone, a leaf, a handful of earth from beneath your feet, or an annoying symptom that won't go away.

Approach whatever comes to you as an aspect of your Self. Sit next to it like a friend. Notice its texture, its smell, its flavor, the sound it makes when you hold it in your hand. Remember that all life is connected.

Once you have integrated this "other" into your being, you will be able to carry its intelligence within you.

When the time is right, ask a question and wait . . . listen for what comes.

Faith

Alchemy is a process of refinement or upgrade organized around the belief that there is something eternal and divine that is an intrinsic part of who you are. This speck of divinity can be refined through art, skill, and practice. It responds to your attention and care, maturing toward the expression of immortal qualities such as wisdom, compassion, courage, serenity, and personal radiance.

Yet, the upgrades or "gold" of alchemy cannot be predicted or forced by the conscious ego, the mind, or will. The cracking of even the most well-crafted and consciously tended vessels is an ever-present possibility. Loss, failure, and death are all possible outcomes of the work. Your job is not to know but rather to trust the process. The work of the will is to faithfully keep bringing you back to the place where miracles can occur—back to your practice, back to the pause, back to the laboratory, back to the relationship, back to cultivating the garden of your life.

Author and environmentalist Derrick Jensen reminds us that we do not stand in front of a tree shouting, "Grow, damn you, grow!" Instead, he references the Greek word *kairos*—the time of destiny or moment of blossoming—to answer the question, "How long does change take?"

Kairos is not under our conscious control. It comes as a kind of grace. All you can do as a person committed to new possibilities for our planet is to keep creating the conditions for change and stay committed to the process. Return again and again to the practice at hand in order for the miracle to occur. In the words of poet Jalāl ad-Dīn Muhammad Rumi, ". . . painstaking work, then the swan spreads its wings."

The Third Key

Pick one small action that you don't do regularly—drinking a cup of tea in silence while watching the sky, feeding sparrows, doing a sun salutation in the morning, writing a note to someone you love or a friend who is estranged, reading something beautiful in the morning. It can be anything.

Decide how long you will continue the practice (a day, one week, one month . . .).

Watch what happens as you work with the practice. Watch your resistance but do it anyway. Watch the tricks you play with yourself to get out of it. Watch the emotions that move through you. Watch your doubt that doing something this simple can make a difference.

And then watch what happens when you do stay with it. Record what you notice in a journal.

Deep Listening

To listen beyond the words, to listen to the spaces between the words, to follow the arc of the emotion all the way to a person's soul . . . this listening is what allows you to recognize the poem, the dream, the riddle, the secret embedded in the story. This attention is what allows you to move beyond the limits of the physical body and enter the sacred space of spirit-level healing.

What distinguishes hearing, an involuntary neurological response to sound waves, from listening, which heals and transforms in an alchemical way?

Listening is a full-body experience that involves all your senses. It is a resonance that constellates between you and another person. It is an exchange of energy. Something comes to life that wasn't there before. I cannot count the number of times a patient has told me, "I feel better just from being heard so deeply. I don't even need needles."

Deep listening is a treatment, a kind of needle that touches the soul. Listening doesn't just happen. It is a practice, a skill that must be developed, cultivated, and honed. Practice the next time someone is telling you something that is difficult to hear. Imagine your heart is an empty bowl of listening. Let words fall into you like drops of Summer rain.

The Fourth Key

In this moment, wherever you are as you read these words, stop and place the tips of your fingers in the slight depression just in front of your ears. In traditional Chinese medicine, this point is called Listening Palace.

Turn your attention to the sounds around you.

Out of this tapestry of sound, find one sound—a voice outside the window, a footfall on a stair, a honking horn, a bird on a branch, a cloud passing, a star falling in a galaxy far away—and offer this sound as a gift to your Heart.

Imaginal Sight

Like the green chlorophyll of the plant kingdom, the human imagination is a converter of light into energy; however, while the chloroplast, the part of the plant that does the converting, transforms sunlight into glucose (chemical energy that fuels metabolic processes and the physical growth of the plant), the imagination transforms spiritual light into images—psychic energy that fuels the psycho-spiritual processes and the soul development of a human being.

In order to work with the light of your imagination, you must learn to work with images, as if seeing in a dream even when you are awake. This way of seeing is not scientific—objective, repeatable, and analytic, but rather alchemical—relational, interactive, and ever-changing. It takes practice. Be patient. What you see with your imaginal sight is determined only by the quality and necessity of the moment, by what is arising now in you and in the people around you.

As it becomes increasingly crucial for people to discern what is "really" going on in the world beyond the superficial and contradictory information from mainstream news sources, to know who and what is life-affirming, and what we need to avoid or confront, this kind of seeing becomes an alchemist's indispensable tool. The following practice will help you to open your inner eyes and bring you back to what ancient alchemists called, the "magick of twilight."

The Fifth Key

Begin by dimming the lights in a room or do this practice at twilight or dawn in a peaceful place.

Find something you want to look at—a tree, a pond, a mountain, a crystal, or even a photo of a person to whom you feel close.

Bring your awareness down into your body. Notice your breath and invite any extraneous thoughts and tensions to drain away.

Notice any tension around your eyes. Squeeze them tightly together and then release them, softening the muscles. Allow your eyes to sink back into the sockets, to rest easily in the hollow of the orbital bones.

Rather than seeing with your eyes, see through them. Invite the outer world to come into you rather than going out to get it.

Do not focus directly on your object. Instead, let your vision wander over, around, and through it. Feel the sensation of the light as it enlivens your optic nerves and settles gently on the folds of your imagination.

Now close your eyes and "see" the object with your inner eyes, the eyes of your imagination. You may see a halo of light begin to form around your object or another image form nearby. You may see a face take shape in the bark of the tree or an entire landscape in the clouds.

If you continue to practice this meditation, taking images from nature into your being and exploring them with your inner sight, you will gradually sharpen the eyes of your imagination and begin to see with your heart what cannot be seen with your ordinary eyes.

Inner Sensing

A river of experience flows through you as you make your way to work, pick up your child from school, stop at the grocery store, or rush to your couple's therapy session. In any given moment of the day, you have a hunch, a feeling, a rush of emotion, but you're too busy to notice. You can't quite hear the messages of your body. You don't know what the hunch, the feeling, the rush of emotion needs. The divine whispers through you, but you don't yet speak its language.

The phone rings and, like a frightened cat, your spine stiffens. You wake in the morning with a heaviness in your chest. Your partner leaves the house and your breath catches; there is something you meant to say, but what?

Alchemists recognize that these mutterings and murmurings of our bodies matter. Our neuromuscular reactions need to be treated with care and regarded as friendly messengers even when they make us uncomfortable. The ripples of qi that surface as the life force moves through us offer direct insight into the needs and desires of our souls.

Inner Sensing is a practice that combines Zen mindfulness and qi gong inner visioning with Eugene Gendlin's Focusing practice. I use Inner Sensing daily. Whether you have a specific issue, problem, or question that you want to work with, or you simply want to get in touch with the wisdom of your body without a specific goal, this practice will help you get closer to your own truth and discover information you need to get closer to your Tao. With practice, Inner Sensing gets easier and you'll learn to hear your body's messages more efficiently, perhaps even in the space of a pause.

The Sixth Key

Begin by reversing the light! Drop your awareness down and in. You can close your eyes or leave them open. Bring awareness to your body and say hello.

Beginning at the top of your head, travel downward, using your imaginal sight to view each part of your body as your awareness drops down from the top of your head to the tips of your toes. Bring an attitude of kindness to any fidgety, painful, or upset feelings you encounter along the way.

Once you've journeyed through your body, invite any tensions, worries, or concerns that you don't need to drop away. If some things want to stick around, make room for them too.

Now, invite your awareness to gather in the area between your pelvis and your chin and feel into what is going on there.

Bring your attention back to this area if it wanders. Rest in this spacious awareness without "doing" for a few moments. The core is home base, a place you can always come back to.

If you have identified an issue that you want to work with, bring it into your awareness. Notice what happens in your core. What tightens? What loosens? How is your breathing? If nothing forms, notice what "nothing" feels like.

If you do not have a specific issue, ask yourself, "How am I doing in there right now?" and notice what comes.

You will become aware of a vague bodily sensation that comes in response to your awareness and interest. The vague sensation is somewhere in between physical and emotional, like the feeling you get in your body when you've forgotten something even though you don't know precisely what you left behind. This bodily sensation is what Eugene Gendlin named the "Body Felt Sense."

The Body Felt Sense doesn't need to make sense to your rational mind. Give it room to be surprising or odd, pleasurable, unfamiliar, confusing.

Ask what the feeling needs or wants you to know. Without rushing, directing, interrupting, or demanding, deeply listen to your body.

When you get what it is your body wants you to know, you will feel a physical shift, a sense of movement, release and relaxation, emotion or a change in your breathing.

Close the process by writing the information you receive down in your journal. If there is an action step you need to take, do it promptly. Don't put it off. This will keep your process alive and moving.

When you practice Inner Sensing, you move between your everyday three-dimensional experience and the multidimensional nonlinear experience of the dream time. In traditional cultures, this movement was a recognized part of all sacred ritual and the end of the ritual was marked by some kind of acknowledgment or gift giving. Appreciate your body by taking a deep breath or gently touching a part of you that needs energy, healing, or warmth. Stretch. Ring a bell. Be grateful.

Prima Materia

In alchemy, every transformation begins with lead—a seemingly immovable, inert, opaque block of darkness, an impasse or chaos. Without this lead, there is no opus, no work, no potential for anything new to come to life.

In Alchemical Healing, transformation begins with a kind of lead, *prima materia*, which means "first matter." It refers to the presenting symptom that begins the work of healing. The prima materia is the problem that finally gets your attention. It is the cipher, the unanswerable question, the intractable pattern. It is the thing that confounds you, stops you in your tracks, engages, enrages, enthralls, or frightens you. It is the bad habit you can't stop, the pain that has no identifiable cause, the recurring dream you do not understand, the deadened relationship you cannot leave, the relentless hope, the unrequited passion, the stuck place that will not shift.

Sometimes, the prima materia is a conglomeration of personal and ancestral stories and shadowy feelings we have buried—the angry, depressed, grieving, introverted parts of ourselves we don't want to feel or look at. One patient described it as "a loneliness that follows me everywhere I go." Another said she felt that the despair of her holocaust-surviving father kept her from her own joy.

The alchemical paradox is that these neglected, rejected parts are our most important allies, the angels who have kept our souls safe until we are able to heal; they are guides to the Self. The prima materia is the raw material of change.

Take a look at your life and consider what you would most like to get rid of. Here is where you will find it—in the headaches, bed bugs, burned toast, births, deaths, failed projects, family fights, love affairs, lost gambles, mismatched socks, stubborn symptoms, and annoying habits that plague your life. Right here. Right now.

The Seventh Key

Use Inner Sensing to get in touch with your body.

Move your awareness from the top of your head all the way down to your feet. If you can't feel your feet, try wiggling each of your toes separately.

Don't try to change anything. Everything is okay as it is. Just check in to see how things are doing down there in the darkness.

Once you have said hello to your body, bring your attention to the area about two inches below your belly button, what Taoist alchemists called the *dantian*, the cinnabar field, the alchemical cauldron of your body. You can place your hands there to help you focus on it. Take a breath down to this part of you. In alchemy, this lower cauldron of the belly is considered one of the main places where renewal and transformation occurs.

Now ask yourself, "What is between me and feeling all okay about my life?" Be honest.

Don't rush the answer but let it come up from your body. At first you might just feel the prima materia as a hazy wordless feeling in your gut. Don't worry, just wait for a few moments and then see if you can find a word or phrase that gets at what you are feeling there and imagine you could move it over to the side of you.

Repeat the question "What is between me and feeling all okay about my life?" and move over the next thing you find.

Keep going with this process until you feel you have nothing left to move.

Take a look at all those parts and pieces of your life that are sitting there right next to you. See which one bothers you most and invite it to the table.

Now sit back and say hello to the most cherished guest at the banquet of your life!

Congratulations! You found your prima materia, the lead you are going to turn into gold. Here is the basis of your inner work. Whether it is big or small, something that has bothered you for a long time, or something that appeared just a moment ago, it's what is present for you now. The problem or symptom is the door you walk through to become who you are fully meant to be. Even if it feels bad or boring or dumb, from an alchemical perspective, this prima materia is a precious treasure in disguise.

As you move through the following chapters, bring the concepts, practices, and tools to bear on your lead. Have patience. Bring courage. In this way, you will make modern-day alchemy a practical part of your life. In this way, you will also master skills and tools that will allow you to help others. In this way, you will join alchemists throughout time and begin the great work of healing and transforming our world.

Chapter 7

Archetypes

In this way was the Universe created. From this comes many wondrous Applications, because this is the Pattern.

—The Emerald Tablet (Precept Six)

Night Vision

I am outside a building on a terrace. It is night. I turn to the right and see a large brown owl sitting at the edge of the terrace looking directly at me. The bird is powerful, mysterious, sitting calmly on its perch on the wall. I think, "I know this owl. I have seen it before, and I have always longed to see it again. Now it is with me."

The owl spreads its wings and flies off into the forest.

Turning slightly to my left, I see on a barren patch of open ground an old beggar woman, a crone, swathed in skirts and veils. The woman is spinning around and around. As she spins, her clothes spread out like black wings. I am afraid of her. I don't want to give her money or interact with her in any way. But then I realize she is in her own world, doing what she needs to do. She does not need my money. She only needs me to know that she is there, spinning in the night. She only needs me to recognize her.

I feel as if something is now accomplished and complete. I watch the woman for a while, then turn and walk home. I hear the whispers of her skirts and veils as the beggar woman spins in the distance and then, above me, the hooting of an owl.

This is a fragment of a dream that I had the year I turned fifty. It marked a significant shift in life focus, a new commitment to my ideas about the soul, and an inner imperative to honor my "night vision"—my ability to see into the mysterious darkness of the body soul, the inner world, and the unconscious, as well as the outer day-light world of the conscious mind. Soon after the dream, I decided to begin teaching and pursue publishing my first book. I also painted the owl. To this day, the wide-eyed night bird sits above my desk and guides me back and forth between the domains of daytime and darkness. This dream preceded a knowing that became conscious gradually, as the years passed, as people I cared for died, as my own physicality, interests, and energies shifted. The owl came to forewarn me of something on the way—the wild weird beauty, the relentless-ness, the potential artistry and liberation of aging; something to be accomplished; and an acceptance of a task: to remember, to witness, to surrender.

The owl dream is just one of hundreds of dreams that I have recorded in my journals plus the hundreds more that patients have shared with me. Dreams of tour buses barreling across the Sinai des-ert, boats floating through Amazonian rivers, teeth peeling layers of shining metallic colors, stolen blue bicycles, church bathrooms, lost car keys, Kansas cyclones, fierce tigers, broken telephones, and an infinite array of houses, trees, dogs and cats, doctors, sandwiches, tsunamis, and cafeterias.

Then there are the images that come from even deeper places, the images that are not personal but universal: concentric circles in the sand, bleached white bones, stone bathtubs, triangular doorways leading into dark caves, babies covered in wet clay, feathered ser-pents, storm clouds, towering trees, springs, crystals, huts, many-storied houses, hallways, mountains, and long roads. Although these images come from the contemporary dreams of my patients and stu-dents, we discover them again in fairy tales and myths as well as the art and poetry of cultures throughout time and space, from Siberia to Mexico, from Tibet to Egypt, from Celtic Ireland to sub-Saharan

Africa. These perennial symbols arise from the deepest layers of our awareness. Like the instincts, they are not taught but are innate and inborn, regenerative and persistent. Like the owl in my dream, we know them from "before." And we know them "after."

Traditional Chinese medicine is filled with these enduring images, as are classical Chinese medical texts, writings of the great Taoist poets, and ancient Chinese myths. Names of acupuncture points like Great Abyss, Spirit Burial Ground, Insect Ditch, Gate of Origin, Celestial Pivot, and hundreds of others call us back to this other world, as do the great Taoist poet Chuang Tzu's stories of belching trees, river lords, sacred turtles, hunchbacks, mudfish, and the eternal phoenix who eats nothing but the rarest fruit and drinks water only from the clearest springs. Master physicians gave illnesses evocative names such as Wind Invasion, Spirit Disturbance, Rising Fire, Possession by Demons, Damp Heat, Running Piglet, and the dreaded and deadly Separation of Yin and Yang. They spoke of symptoms like plum pits stuck in the throat or the desire to climb tall towers and tear off one's clothes while singing. Pulses feel like tight wires, soggy threads, or pearls rolling in a bowl of water.

When I first began talking to my patients in the language of the ancient Chinese, I expected that there would be a lot of explaining to do. Instead, I was amazed at how readily people accepted and responded to the poetry of a world they had never experienced, had not studied, and could not consciously understand. Almost without exception, patients made significant connections between the poetic images and their issues, symptoms, and healing processes. It was as if they were being offered something precious that they had been waiting for, a way to talk about their physical and emotional symptoms that elevated them from annoying inconveniences, medical expenses, or frightening disabilities to experiences with their own unique story, meaning, and possibly even purpose.

Without any previous training in Chinese medicine, my patients responded to the point names, resonated with the myths, and related in direct, embodied ways to yin and yang in their own lives. I found that using language and the imagination to bring these ideas and images into a treatment had an effect on physiology. Similarly, introducing myths and mythical beings enlivened the treatment and helped my patients reconnect to forgotten parts of their own being. I saw that the Red Bird of the Heart, the White Tiger of the Lungs, the Dark Goddess *Xi Wang Mu*, or the Blue-Black Tortoise who guards the Gate of Life at the base of the spine lived not only in ancient China but also in our modern Western souls.

I noticed the same sense of recognition, visceral response, and acceptance when I brought in images drawn from astrology, yoga, shamanism, flower essence therapy, dream work, and many other ancient healing traditions. I asked myself how these images, symbols, and myths from completely different times and cultures could inspire such curiosity, appreciation, and easy receptivity in modern Western patients. Why did it feel so important to bring these images into the treatment room? What was unique about the healing that happened in this atmosphere?

What is an Archetype?

Pieces fell into place for me when I read about C. G. Jung's early twentieth century investigations into a related phenomenon in his clinical practice in Switzerland. Jung repeatedly found correlations between images in his patients' dreams and visions—snakes biting their own tails, squares within circles, or upside-down trees—and images he discovered in ancient alchemical drawings, myths, and aboriginal art. In almost all cases, there was no way that the patients could have known that their dream images were mirrored in an ancient Egyptian alchemical scroll, a Taoist text, or an African shaman's prayer shawl. Yet the parallels were unmistakable. Jung was fascinated and intrigued by the "[a]nalogy, sometimes even identity, between the various myth motifs and symbols" and his patients' fantasies and visions.

One of Jung's crucial breakthroughs in understanding came through a schizophrenic patient's hallucinatory image of a long phallic-shaped tube that extended down from the sun. The patient claimed that the tube's motion caused the winds to blow on Earth and "[w]hen he moved his head from side to side, the sun's phallus moved with it, and that was where the wind came from." Soon after working with this patient, Jung came across almost exactly the same image in a second-century Egyptian papyrus, the *Mithras Liturgy*, which had been translated into German. The Liturgy described a tube that hangs down from the sun and is the origin of the wind. This tube veers from East to West and generates wind corresponding to its movements.

The "coincidental" parallel of his patient's vision with the description in the ancient papyrus led Jung to a startling conclusion: his patient's hallucinations, rather than being singular random outpourings of a deranged mind, were the result of a breaking down of individual ego identity that catapulted him into a deep and primal level of awareness not ordinarily available to modern waking consciousness. Jung came to understand that this deeper sector of the psyche is a vast reservoir of universal, primordial images that exert a powerful influence on all human beings throughout space and time. These images well up through the layers of the psyche to appear in art, dreams, religious rituals, drug-induced hallucinations, myths, and fairy tales as well as in the psychotic visions of schizophrenics. Like the instincts, the images are innate, an intrinsic part of the human psyche and nervous system dating back to our earliest beginnings. And like the instincts, they have a powerful capacity to protect us, move us, propel us forward into life, possess us, and also help us heal and grow.

Through his encounter with this psychotic patient as well as his ongoing study of the dreams and visions of other patients, Jung recognized the importance of this deep reservoir of ancestral images to understand the human psyche both in its pathology and its health. He came to view it as a primal psychic system of a universal and impersonal nature that does not develop through our historical encounters with family, culture, or education, but is inborn, inherited from our earliest ancestors. Due to its commonality among all human beings, Jung called this domain of the psyche the "collective unconscious" to distinguish it from the personal unconscious. He viewed it as the link between individual awareness, instinctual life, and the vast bewilderment of the cosmos. He called the primordial images that arise from these psychic depths "archetypes" and felt that they connected us not only to the roots of our being but also to the divine creative energy of the universe.

Archetypes are hints to riddles the conscious mind alone could never answer. They are less "things" than living tendencies, open channels where psychic energy flows. They point us in a direction. C. G. Jung borrowed the word *archetype* from the Greek to refer to the significant symbols and patterns he came across repeatedly in the dreams of his patients and the art, myths, and religious texts of the ancient civilizations he was exploring. *Arche* means "first" or "origin" and *typos* means "mark, blow, or impression." For the Greeks, the word had to do with how being came from nonbeing, how the forms of the world emerged from the formless void, how the unity of ideal perfection is reflected in the infinite, imperfect multiplicity of the world.

The archetypes are the contents of the collective unconscious. They are embedded in the threads of our DNA, impressed into the subtle body like a blow, an indelible mark, a block of type pressed down onto the pages of the soul. These images are as much a part of our makeup as our arms and legs, as the capacity of our lungs to breathe, and our hearts to beat. Just as the physical structures of our bodies begin to organize from the moment of conception, these images also begin to impress themselves on our psyches *a priori*— before we even come to be. They organize our way of entering into our life and our way of leaving it. They are an intrinsic part of our nature as humans, just as fundamental, irrepressible, and necessary to our survival as our inborn animal instincts.

The outer expression of an archetype changes according to time, culture, and individual experience, but its fundamental structure does not. Just as a robin's nest will have the same form and function whether it is woven in an elm tree in Kensington Garden or a spruce tree in the woods of Maine, an archetype will retain its essential nature, function, and drive wherever it appears. For example, the Goddess of Love may show herself as Aphrodite in Greece, Venus in Rome, Isis in Egypt, Oshun in Africa, a woman emerging from a fluted sea shell in an Italian Renaissance painting, or Marilyn Monroe in the modern cinema, but in all her infinite guises she retains her fertile sensuality, potent sexual desire, and feminine allure. She seduces us into the madness of love, the complexity of relationship, the joys and burdens of procreation, and the risky uncertain business of life itself.

Archetypes are channels or conduits into which our psychic energy, emotions, and behavioral responses naturally flow. A healthy human infant, for example, comes into life with the outline or space for "mother"—the mother archetype—already in it. It is ready to be held, nurtured, and nursed before it ever meets its human caregiver. It is born with a knowing of mother in its bones, blood, fingertips, and taste buds. This Body Felt Sense knowing of mother exists deep in its being and allows it to spontaneously recognize, trust, and respond to its care-giving parent as long as the real and the archetypal are sufficiently close in quality and behavior. Throughout our lives, long after our biological mother has passed away, this innate a priori mother continues to live in us, directing and supporting us, arising at times as a longing, a comfort, a loss, as the warm furry body of a dog in a dream, a green mountain or a warm pond, a table filled with food and flowers, a good sleep after a long journey, or a lover's nurturing embrace.

The concept of the archetypes opened a doorway for me and my practice. It allowed me to make sense of the immediacy of my patients' responses to the images and poetry of traditional Chinese medicine. It helped me understand the healing potency of these images and how they influence the healing process simply by bringing them into the treatment room. It helped me understand why images, myths, and poetry transcend time and culture as well as how they could shift an experience from the everyday world of mental consciousness to another domain where body and soul, physical and psychological, seamlessly intertwine. Through this shift, something happened in the room that was unexpected and powerful, that took the treatment beyond stress reduction, energy balancing, health maintenance, or symptomatic fix to an experience of personal renewal.

Conscious use of the archetypes allowed me to bridge the gap between the world of ancient China and the modern Western consciousness of the patients I work with. Over time, I came to recognize archetypes as powerful tools, another kind of needle, that I could intentionally use to move qi, open channels, and support a patient's journey toward their own healing and wholeness, toward their Tao. Eventually, I came to see work with archetypes as an intrinsic part of Alchemical Healing.

Filling in an Empty Archetype

You come into the world with archetypes already embedded in your nervous system. You are born with a space in your soul for Mother. Father. Sister. Brother. Friend. Healer. Hero. Mentor. And you are born ready to meet the people who will reflect these universal qualities back to you as personal, limited, embodied expressions of something divine. If the outer people and conditions you encounter through the various stages of life are adequately close in kind and quality to the archetypes already waiting within, you meet them, integrate them, and these qualities gradually become a part of your creative and functional self. Archetype becomes identity.

Child psychologist D. W. Winnicott devoted his life to the painstaking observation of infant development. He was particularly struck by the child's critical need for what he came to call the "good enough mother." He discovered that what human beings most need in order to grow into self-confident, generous, functional adults is not a perfect mother. In fact, because it is impossible for a human being to exactly replicate an archetype, striving for that kind of perfection gets in the way. Winnicott found that the most basic human need is for a caregiver who brings just enough of the archetypal maternal qualities of warmth, nurturance, and reliable presence to "stand in" for the archetype until those qualities come to life as a part of a child's developing self.

But what happens when the outer person isn't "good enough"? What if the mother is suffering from depression after the death of a previous child and cannot express warmth? What if the older sibling has a severe illness and cannot be relied on as a companion? What if the mentor betrays the sacred bonds of trust through boundary violations or envy?

When the "real person" does not resonate adequately with the archetype, the process of healthy development breaks down. In my practice, I see it as a hole in a patient's soul that is as painful and debilitating on a psychic level as a festering wound on the body. I have seen this psychic wounding manifest as a terrible gnawing hunger, an insatiable longing, a hopelessness, or a nameless rage. Until the wound heals, it usually requires constant self-medicating and numbing in the form of dissociation and various forms of addictive behavior. And yet in this lead there lies the gold. The place of wounding is also the place where the healing begins. In the realm of archetypes, the hole contains the wholeness.

As a result of our work together, James gradually became aware of a feeling that no one had his back when he needed to speak in public or act as an authority. The feeling of "backlessness" left him anxious, shaky, doubting his self-worth, and hesitant to take on personal or professional risks. The situation led to his sense of being stuck in a job he disliked, with few friends and no close intimacy.

Over several months, we worked with acupuncture to move qi through a meridian in James's back called the Governing Vessel that enlivens yang qi and strengthens the backbone. He took Larch flower essence, which restores self-confidence and supports a feeling of powerful verticality that mirrors the upright shape of the larch tree. But it was during a process of Inner Sensing when he recognized that the empty feeling at his back was the hole where his father should have been.

James's parents divorced when he was ten years old. After the divorce, he lived with his mother and rarely saw his father, who had always been distant but after the divorce disappeared almost completely. Of his mother, James said, "I knew she would always be there. I knew she loved me. And that's great. That's beautiful. But still, I always felt there was something important missing."

He realized that not having a father around, especially as he was entering puberty and trying to figure out how to be a man in the world, left him with a big emptiness, a hole that he was always afraid of falling into. And yet, when he turned his gaze to that hole in our session, there was something there, something that made him smile.

I asked if he could imagine this father who would be the right match, the right guy, the right chemistry. He paused and then he nodded his head, emphatically, yes. I asked James to describe what this person would be like.

> A good father is someone you grow up with, someone you know over time. You get to watch him handle adversity, challenges that come up and you see that, no matter what, he stays the same person. He doesn't get all turned around when things get tough. He hangs in. He stays. Not like my actual father. I mean, when I think about people I know, I can't really think of anyone. I guess I'm going to have to create him inside of me. That's the father I want to become. That's the father I am going to be.

Working with Archetypes

In Alchemical Healing, archetypes are used in much the same way that an acupuncturist uses needles, as tools to move qi, access the life force, and support the opening of stuck places in transformational processes. They can also be used as filters or nets through which you access and gather potent transpersonal cosmic energies and step them down sufficiently to be safely worked with in your life. In addition, archetypes form the basis of the imaginal practices and meditations of alchemy. They are key components in astrology, dream work, and the Inner Sensing practice introduced in the last chapter. Psychologically, archetypes can be understood as self-generated energies that propel you toward your own survival, growth, and development.

From the perspective of alchemists and magicians of earlier eras, archetypes are spirits, autonomously functioning divine soul beings with their own perceptions, drives, insights, and desires. They are messengers who link humans to the divine. They come in an infinite array of costumes and disguises, as wily tricksters, wise teachers, fierce opponents, long-lost lovers. They live in the betwixt and between of the psyche, "part of us" yet also separate.

Whether you view them as images, principles, or living spirits, it is unwise to underestimate the power and purpose of the archetypes. Just as the instincts irresistibly compel us toward biological preservation and growth, the archetypes propel us forcibly toward our psychospiritual development and personal evolution. They come in service to your entelechy, your innate drive to become the fullest possible expression of your innate nature.

Even when you are not aware of them, archetypes move you. They grab you in the gut, inspire you, heal you, and call you back to yourself in new ways. Even when you do not know they are there, you are affected and touched by their presence. Whether or not you relate consciously to the power of the King archetype, for example, you are affected when the president is knowingly deceitful or a beloved world leader dies. You respond with relief and joy when Simba wins the battle over his manipulative, death-mongering uncle Scar and restores fertility, peace, and hope to the Pride Lands in Disney's *Lion King*.

Archetypes inform the shape of our myths, our creative impulses, and our relationships. They beckon to us from movie screens. They appear as faces peering out at us from the bark of trees, babies smiling at us from grocery carts, handsome strangers, and round gleaming stones picked from tide pools. Whenever you are dazzled, grabbed, arrested, compelled, wandering, lost, late, or blind to your own reason, you can suspect that an archetype is present and has something important to tell you. It is imperative that you slow down, breathe, recognize its presence, and listen carefully.

Recognizing Their Presence

You know an archetype is present not through your mind but through your body and your emotions. You feel a primal, instinctual energy come into your life, something entrances, seduces, attracts, repels, confuses. You fall in love with the fireman who rescued your cat from the roof of the house. You can't stop watching the royal wedding on television. You blow up at your mother-in-law every time she calls.

Your jaw clenches when you hear the word *priest*, or you feel anxiety creeping up your spine at the sight of a cemetery. Notice how the energy shifts when you read the words *Republican, liberal, immigrant, homeland, black,* and *white*.

Mother, father, lover, child—you feel these experiences as a tug of emotion, a rush of anger, a driving desire, an inexplicable fear, disorientation, or longing. The response surprises you. You feel it in your throat, your chest, your churning stomach, the heady rush of excitement throughout your entire body, the compelling need to say something you already know you will regret or an unexpected loss of words.

When you are in the presence of archetypal energy, it is as if a powerful tide is pulling you away from your individual identity into the vast depths of the collective unconscious. You are drawn into fits of melodrama, pits of depression, flights of grandiosity. You make impetuous purchases, run stop signs, and enter into ridiculous love affairs. Jungian analyst Harry Wilmer describes these experiences of insanity in ordinarily sane people as "[b]eing in the clutches of an archetype." We are in their grip and they hold us captive with a power that we often cannot control.

As an acupuncturist I think of "being in the clutches of an archetype" as an energy block. Like a block, it is a place where qi or life force gets arrested, bottled up, and out of reach of conscious awareness, but it is also a place of potential vitality, an entryway to a new possibility. Seeing and acknowledging an archetype block is like needling the right point at the right time so that your life force can begin to flow again.

Archetypes are paradoxical, and similar to the medicine that cures in small doses and kills in large doses, they need to be approached with caution, respect, and gratitude. Most of all, they need to be recognized and related to so that their potentially destructive "larger than life" energies can be titrated through the filter of consciousness. Welcome and sit next to the archetypes that arrive on your doorstep but resist the impulse to become identified with them. This prevents you from becoming an unconscious conduit of their energies, but instead allows you to get closer to their wisdom and tap into their renewing reservoir of life-giving transpersonal energy.

> Begin by paying attention to how your Body Felt Sense changes in response to certain words, people, and situations.
>
> When you notice an unusual bodily shift, an impulse to react with an outburst of emotion or hurtful words, an overwhelming attraction, take a breath and pause! Pause . . . breathe . . . remember . . . ask yourself when you have felt this feeling before. What does it remind you of?
>
> Use Inner Sensing to feel into the nature of your body response. What is its color, its texture, its emotion? Why is it coming? What does it need? What qualities are present?
>
> Is there a public figure, movie star, television personality, book character, or someone you know that reminds you of how you feel in this reactive state? Give the Body Felt Sense a name and get ready to relate to it!

Relating to Archetypes

Benjamin and I got a powerful lesson in the importance of listening carefully to archetypes that show up in relationship when, after sixteen years of knowing each other, we finally made the decision to legally marry. We had carefully weighed the outer social, political, and economic ramifications of our decision. We waited until it looked likely that gay marriage would be legalized in Maine (the people of Maine voted in the bill two months after our ceremony) so that the LGBTQ+ members of our community shared the same rights to legalize and publicly celebrate the commitment. We spoke to our lawyer and sorted out the complexities of shared resources and inheritance in our blended family. We had a budget and a date. We were ready to go.

But we hadn't reckoned with the inner situation and the power of the *coniunctio*—the archetype of the divine marriage. Weddings have a potent force field, and soon all our friends had something to say about it. Some expressed shock and dismay that after so many years of standing for some alternative expression of relationship, we'd made what they viewed as a conventional decision. Others were excited and wanted to help. Our friends were more than generous with everything from their time to their organizational skills to the tablecloths, napkins, and china we'd use for the reception. A farmer friend offered a lamb and two others said they'd take care of the outdoor grill. Soon, everyone had gotten involved.

Rings. Clothes. The DJ, the cake, chairs, and tables. Everything was falling into place. It was all going so well except that every time Benjamin and I sat down to do some planning, we started fighting. It was as if a nasty grumpy ghoul was doing everything in its power to ruin the party. It got so bad and we were hating each other so much at one point that we came close to calling the whole thing off. But then we remembered, took a pause, and turned our attention inward.

When we tuned in to the field between us—the feelings and atmosphere that constellated when we actually sat down together—we felt a sadness, a resentment, and a loneliness. The space was heavy and musty like a house that had been closed up for a very long time. Opening to my imaginal sight, I saw a child in tattered clothes sitting alone in an empty room while everyone was happily busy elsewhere. When we asked the child why it had shown up right when we were getting married, it didn't have a lot to say. But when we stayed with it, we recognized that the archetype of the abandoned child that was present in both our personal life stories had taken over our relationship. It became clear to us that in the midst of all the extroverted excitement and planning, we had abandoned our own relational connection.

After that, we started to carve out time for the inner aspects as well as the outer logistics of our wedding. We took the writing of our vows seriously. We checked in with each other's feelings and made space for our fears of intimacy and commitment as well as our hopes for deepening connection. I grappled with the feelings of grief in knowing that my mother and brother, who had both recently died, would not be present to celebrate with us. Benjamin struggled to make peace with the complex feelings he had regarding his decision to exclude most members of his family at the event. We tried to remember that every aspect of the ceremony had an inner symbolic resonance that needed to be respected. We kept coming back to our commitment to each other's healing and spiritual development as well as our shared commitment to our friends, our community, and the world. Gradually, the archetype of the abandoned child transformed into the divine child who is the carrier of new life and new possibilities.

The wedding took place in the field by our home and the reception in a rickety nearby barn. It was a wild conglomeration of family and friends old and new. The early Autumn rays of sun broke through the silver clouds just as we took our vows. The ceremony went beautifully. The food was great, and everyone danced all night. But I have absolutely no doubt that none of that would have mattered if we hadn't taken the time to listen in to the ragged angel, the abandoned child who had come to call us back to ourselves and to one another.

Making It Real: Ritual and Practice

In order to bring the spiritual potency of an archetype into your life, you have to find a way to bring it down to Earth. Grounding your work through ritual is one of the best ways to make the archetype a part of your world, to make it conscious and real, and at the same time, honor its unknowable divinity. It is also a way to actualize the changes that the archetype is urging you toward.

A ritual is a physical act that grounds a psychological insight or spiritual revelation in form, word, and action. It is one of the most efficient expressions of magical consciousness. When Benjamin and I turned our attention to writing our wedding vows, we engaged in a ritual that honored the divinity of the child who had come to us. Touching an acupuncture spirit point, applying an essential oil, placing a flower in a glass vase with intention, and hanging a prism in a sunny window are other relatively simple ways to honor the archetypes on a daily basis.

Archetypes need your attention. They need your devotion, interest, and care in order to manifest their potent healing and life-giving effects in the world. When you neglect their hunger, wisdom, desires, and needs, they keep coming at you from the outside in perplexing and annoying ways that stall the forward movement of your life. But when you attend to them, honor them, and make space for them, they become healing allies and trusted guides to the sacred country of the soul.

Chapter 8

Turning the Wheel of Life

Every living thing and every person on the planet is a unique embodiment and combination of the five Elements.

—J. R. Worsley, *Classical Five-Element Acupuncture*

Agents of Transformation

Our word *season* is an incantation, an invocation, and a prayer. *Season* is born from the Latin word *satio*, which refers to the time of seed sewing. For traditional cultures, the great round of the seasons—Spring, Summer, Late Summer, Autumn, and Winter—corresponds directly with the phases of the vegetative cycle. The seasonal shifts of darkness and light, sunshine and rain, warmth and coolness, determine the timing of changes on our planet—the sprouting of the seed, the blossoming of the flower, the harvesting of the fruit, and the decaying of organic matter. Even now, our food sources as well as our survival depend on this rhythmic movement and its relationship to the cycles of birth, growth, life, and death. Deep in the magical, mythical layers of our consciousness, we recognize that each season brings forth its own alchemy. Each has its own gift. Each carries a piece of our soul in the lining of its cloak.

Every season reflects an archetype, an imprint we recognize. Ancient Taoist alchemists based an entire philosophy and healing system on this cycle of change. They called this system *wu xing*, the Five Elements. Today, the medicine based on this system is referred to as Five Element Acupuncture. British osteopath J. R. Worsley is credited with first bringing the Five Elements to the attention of the Western world in the early 1970s. He reminds us that, "The Elements are alive both around us and in us; they describe the movement of all life and all energy and embody all the qualities which we encounter in Nature. Through understanding the five Elements we may begin to understand both Nature and ourselves."

In this system, each phase of the yearly cycle, each footprint or Element, brings together a family of many different yet related ideas—seasonal correspondences, vegetative phases, colors, sounds, and energetic associations. Each Element relates to an emotion, an acupuncture meridian and set of acupuncture points, specific organs as well as textures, and atmospheres and flavors of life experience. Each one is a unique and invaluable agent of change. And each one is a part of you.

In order to access the healing power of wu xing, you will need to open to nature and the synchronous, symbolic wisdom of magical and mythical awareness. You are invited to become like the "healers of old" who knew the subtlety of the world directly through their enlivened senses. The Five Element Wheel has been continuously in use as a form of diagnosis and treatment for the past 2,500 years, and it is still available to support you in transforming your inner as well as your outer world.

The Wheel of Life

The Elements are symbolic expressions of change through time. Water becomes Wood. Wood becomes Fire. The cyclic movement through the five phases describes the dynamic succession of life processes in nature and in you.

If you spend time meditating on the symbol of the Circle and the Pentacle, you will see that movement through the Five Elements follows two different paths:

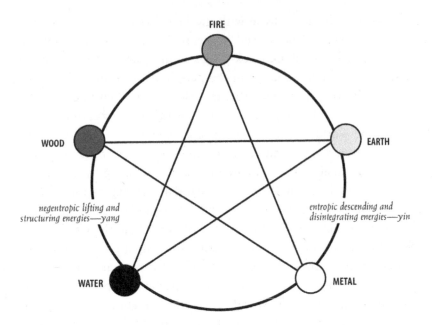

Figure 9. The Five Element Wheel

The *sheng* Life or Generative Cycle moves clockwise around the
outer circle. One element generates and nurtures the next;
for example, Water generates Wood, Wood generates Fire,
etc. The energy on the left side of the circle is yang and
negentropic. It resists the pull of gravity and moves upward
toward growth and expansion. The energy on the right side
of the circle is yin and entropic. It surrenders to gravity
and moves downward toward dissolution, contraction, and
darkness.

The *k'o* Limiting or Qualifying Cycle moves from Wood to
Earth, Earth to Water, Water to Fire, Fire to Metal, Metal
to Wood. One element limits, refines, and leaves a legacy
for the element located across from it on the pentacle; for
example, Water qualifies the nature of Fire, Fire qualifies the
nature of Metal, etc.

I have studied and lived with the Five Element Wheel for more than thirty years. I have used it personally to understand my own creative work, to unlock stuck places in my soul, and to encourage positive growth and change in the people close to me. I have used it clinically to support my patients. I also use it when I need a more expansive view of how processes are unfolding in our current culture and in the world. From my own lived experience, I would say that this deceptively simple alchemical map describes the cycle of growth and change in all of carbon-based life, in every being with a soul.

The Five Element Wheel is a mandala, an expression of unity in diversity, a geometric pattern that offers a glimpse of the divine order in the universe. It is also a symbol of the Self, the wholeness of an individual personality, and the authentic impulse to become what is foundational to every human life. Our lives are an expression of this cosmic wheel as we move from the gestational power of Water, the initiating impulse of Wood, through the maturation of Fire, the ripening of Earth, the letting go of Metal, and back again to the deep rest and regeneration of Water, not just once but repeatedly throughout our lives.

As you engage with the material of this chapter and deepen your familiarity with the Elements, you'll recognize parts of yourself reflected back to you through this lens. At the end of each section, you will find clues and questions that will help identify what role each Element plays in your prima materia as well as the "elemental gold" hidden within your current lead. Your assessment will help you determine which medicinals, acupuncture pressure points, archetypes, and meditation practices you might choose to call on and explore as part of your continuing Alchemical Healing.

Spinning the Wheel

We enter the Wheel of Life in the yin secrecy of Water. Water naturally goes to the low, dark, and hidden places where life originates—the ocean, the womb, the black soil. Water is home base, the bottom, the beginning of a cycle that has no exact beginning and no end.

Water: Gestation

Winter/Seed

Water is related to Winter, the season of hibernation, contraction, and rest, the time when the force of life and the energy to sustain it must be carefully stored and treasured. The fallen seeds and decomposed micronutrients of Autumn are buried beneath the snow. In the womb of the soil, life waits in a state of nearly inert stillness, gestating and gathering strength as it prepares for re-emergence.

Contraction/Expansion/Fear/Courage

Water comes just after the lowest point in the wheel when the cycle reaches its turning point and begins its ascension skyward. Water represents the moment when night, cold, compression, darkness, and death reach their furthest extreme and yang qi rises spontaneously from the yin.

The emotion associated with Water is said to be Fear. Fear relates to the survival drives that arise from the depths of our being and our most primal neurological responses to the risks of embodiment. When you feel the vital "fight, flight, or freeze" responses of your adrenals, you are experiencing the paradoxical nature of Water. It can take the form of an icy constricting, contracting, and paralyzing withdrawal. But it can also express as a steamy high-grade energy that propels you forward into assertive, courageous action; an irresistible urge to emerge, to birth, to reach upward and out. So, courage, the opposite of Fear, is also a quality of Water.

Alchemy: Transforming Will into Wisdom

Water calls you to align your individual personal will—your drives, desires, and ambitions—with the greater will of Tao. You sacrifice pushing and the amphetamine-like high of adrenal cortisol and learn to listen deeply to the song of your bodily instincts. In honoring the Water, you spend an hour doing restorative yoga instead of running five miles in the Winter rain. Rather than ratcheting up your nervous system watching the late-night news, you take a warm balsam fir bath. And instead of mourning the loss of youth and the inevitability of death, you discover the serenity, liberation, and wisdom of aging.

Rather than waste precious essences fighting against the way things are, Water invites us to receive life's lessons and to trust the cosmic paradox: with sleep there will be waking and with death there will be a rebirth. Whether we accept the invitation or not, like stones slowly pitted and grooved by a flowing river, our resistances to Water's ultimate dissolving and transforming power will eventually be worn away by the inevitable coursing of time.

Discovering Water Within You

Is your personal will in integrity and alignment with your time, your age, your Tao?

Your lead:

- You feel dry, brittle, shaky, unrooted, and insecure.

- You are exhausted from trying to control the uncontrollable.

- You push yourself beyond your own limits and ignore your body's need for rest.

Your gold:

- You trust not knowing and recognize the value of silence and rest; you lean back into Tao.

- You endure, wait, and gestate until the right moment arises.

- You listen to your body and accept the passage of time and live in alignment with your authentic nature.

Deep in Winter, the sap turns in the unseen roots of the trees. Deep in the seed, desire, curiosity, and courage awaken. As the Wheel turns from Water to Wood, the moment comes when the seed splits, the egg cracks, the water breaks, and birth becomes imperative. Have you rested long enough and been restored by Water's deep resources? Are your roots strong enough to support your branches? Do you have what you need to take the risk of emergence?

Wood: Imagination

Spring/Sprout

Wood is related to Spring, the season of birth, expansion, and growth. The sprout of life thrusts upward to break through the surface of the soil, determined to find its own dream, its own direction, its own pathway. The spirit of this Element is evident in the first blade of green grass that pushes up through the hard, cold ground in late March—rousing, resolute, vigorous, and direct.

Force/Growth/Anger/Hope

Wood represents the bold assertion of the Self as well as the capacity to have a vision for where the Self is going. Wood's direction is upward and outward. This expansiveness is driven by Wood's imperative to grow and become the fullest possible expression of itself.

Wood represents the young, lusty, unimpeded drive of the Self toward its own actualization. We see it clearly in the infamous "No!" of the two-year-old and the unruly rebelliousness of the teenager, where it functions as a way to stake out and affirm the edges of identity. Anger, the emotion associated with Wood, arises when this innately healthy and life-affirming drive is impeded or blocked. When Wood's vision and growth direction is unsupported by other beings, challenged by environmental conditions, or denied by inner psychological holding patterns, it shows up as frustration, rage, irritability, depression, and hopelessness.

Alchemy: Transforming Selfishness into Benevolence

Wood is related to birth and growth, but it is also related to the blueprint of life, the aspect of Tao that informs the unfolding of living structures. When the seed germinates in the dark depths of Water, the Wood Element is already planning its ultimate form, function, and direction toward the sky.

The Wood must be determined and directed to carry out its function as the manifesting agent of possibility. It must have a kind of adolescent self-centeredness. But it must also have fluidity and flexibility to adapt to the needs of others as well as the environment.

In this way, Wood's "Get out of my way!" transforms into "I grow and become my Self in a way that supports the benevolence, justice, and well-being of the Whole."

Science has shown that trees are generous social creatures. Trees feed and heal each other, pool resources, and share water. In his book *The Overstory*, author and eco-activist Richard Powers writes, "If we could understand green, we'd learn how to grow all the food we need in layers three deep . . . with plants that protected one another from pests and stress. If we knew what green wanted, we wouldn't have to choose between the Earth's interests and our own. They'd be the same!"

Discovering Wood Within You

Are you growing and developing toward your ultimate purpose and destiny?

Your lead:

- You feel irritable and unreasonable, aggressive and impatient as if you are constantly banging your head against closed doors.

- If your Wood is depleted, undernourished, and weak, you feel timid and unable to speak up for yourself, endlessly vacillating instead of making clear decisions about small details or large life plans.

- Your imaginal eyes cannot see and there is no hope for the future.

Your gold:

- You have a clear vision and direction for your life; you go to your own edges and stay on track.

- You dream and imagine in creative ways and are able to plan and organize your time in order to manifest your vision.

- You know where you begin and end—you know your boundaries and are able to appropriately affirm them while also benefitting others around you.

In the exuberance of Spring, the tree already knows it will give its life back to the Fire. As the Wheel turns from Wood to Fire, the stem must be strong enough to support the blossom. Have you been directed enough to grow a self that has something to sacrifice? Is your "no" loud enough to support your "yes"? Do you know who you are enough to relate to another? Do you have what you need to open your heart to love?

Fire: Relationship

Summer/Blossom

The Fire Element is related to the season of Summer, the time of year when the solar forces of heat, sunlight, and growth are at their peak. The energetic of this Element is expressed by the blossoming flower that is lifted skyward by the urgent desire to be admired, enjoyed, and pollinated. The flower's seductive beauty, elegant yet fragile structure, indomitable spirit, and anti-gravitational expansive nature tell us a great deal about the Fire Element as it lives within our own souls.

Rising/Clinging/Relationship/Joy

The Fire Element presides at the top of the Wheel, at the point where the life cycle reaches greatest negentropy. Fire comes when the yin forces of entropy, darkness, weight, and gravity have the least influence and the yang energies of growth, heat, and expansion have reached their fullest expression. Its presence marks the moment when the cycle comes closest to Heaven, to the scintillant realms of the sun, the moon, and the stars. For this reason, the Fire Element is associated with the yang, ephemeral Heavenly aspect of the divine, the shen spirit you see in the eyes of a healthy person.

Fire's yang nature is to rise and yet it needs something yin, such as wood, to cling to in order to sustain its burning and flickering upward movement. So, the Fire Element describes the domain of relationship and communication. It regulates the heat and coolness, intimacy and distance, vulnerability and protectiveness of your connections with yourself and with others.

Joy, the Emotion associated with Fire, has a rising and falling quality similar to everything we associate with Fire. In health, the Emotion of Fire expresses a modulated warmth, a happiness that gracefully comes and goes in response to conditions, a stable flame that flickers but is not extinguished. Out of balance, it can show up as hysteria, mania, romantic obsession, a desperate grasping at happiness, or a flatness that completely annihilates relatedness. In order to remain in balance with this emotion, you must accept the natural oscillations of intimacy and distance without clinging. You must stay present to the reality that with each rise, there will be a fall; with each connection, a loss. This practice is the inner alchemy of the Heart that creates the enduring flame of embodied Spirit.

Alchemy: Modulating the Heat

In order for the Fire Element to fulfill its promise for awakening through intimacy, its impetuous flame must be tempered by Water's wisdom and subjected to the limits of right timing and right relationship. Whether you are creating a work of art, birthing an idea, or cultivating a therapeutic encounter, a community, a love affair, a friendship, or your own inner spiritual development, Fire must be modulated to meet the current need.

Images of vessels cracking over a blazing flame are common in alchemical texts. The contrasting image is of a mother hen patiently sitting on her eggs, keeping them just warm enough so that they hatch of their own accord. The brooding hen is a powerful alchemical image and it applies especially to the delicate heat of love in all its myriad manifestations.

Discovering Fire Within You

How are you doing with expressing your true self in your life and in your relationships?

Your lead:

- You experience trembling, erratic emotional instability and an inability to hold steady in a relationship; you rush in and out of intimacy.

- You do not take the time to listen to the messages of your Heart; you do not honor your own intuition.

- You do not pay attention to feelings of invasion; you do not keep yourself safe by setting appropriate boundaries.

Your gold:

- You communicate clearly and authentically, in connection to what you are feeling.

- You feel and modulate your passion, excitement, and enthusiasm without squelching it.

- You appropriately protect and open your heart; you receive the warmth of love and relationship without losing the connection to yourself.

The fleeting moment of high Summer arrives with a sudden surprising clamor of color and then, almost before you catch a glimpse of the ecstatic beauty, it begins to soften and fade under the influence of the yin. The flower petals fall and the ovule begins to grow heavy and swell to form the seeds and fruits that become the harvest of Late Summer. At the peak moment of Fire's blossoming comes the first intimation of compassion and gracious giving that leads to Earth's abundant generosity. Have you made space for your own seductiveness, for the pleasures and the beauty of life? Have you established a balance between self and other? Do you love yourself enough to nurture another?

Earth: Material

Late Summer/Fruit

Like the season of Late Summer to which it is related, the Earth Element is associated with ripening and gathering; with harvest, repletion, and plenty; and with the enjoyment of the products of our creativity, the flourishing of our labor. Earth's vegetative expression is the fruit of the vine, the parts of plants and trees where the capacity to sustain and nourish life is produced and gathered.

Spreading/Embracing/Coagulating/Sympathy

The Earth Element comes at a point on the sheng cycle when life energy tips over the edge of its most extreme upward movement. The downward pull of gravity increases as the negentropic energies of Water, Wood, and Fire decrease. As we move from the left to the right side of the Wheel, there is more yin, more moisture, more matter, more weight, and the dynamic catalyzing energies of the yang are limited by the formative and fixing tendencies of the yin. The limiting of yang spirit by yin matter coagulates, contracts, and transforms the exuberant creativity of Fire into the generous, nourishing bounty of Earth.

This energetic orb is where the enlivening spiritual vitality of the food we eat is transformed into matter and action in the world. Qi takes the form of muscle, movement, intention, and prayer and our ideas and visions bear the slow, devoted, and sometimes tedious process of becoming grounded in reality.

The Emotion is Sympathy, a spreading out and giving of the self that allows us to feel for another and, like the Earth, nourish and support those we care for.

Alchemy: Transforming Sympathy into Empathy

Throughout history, humans have associated the archetype of the Divine Mother as well as the nurturing, sustaining, protecting aspects of the personal mother with the fertile and nourishing capacities of the Earth. However, just as the Earth can become arid and unproductive, the Mother can also withhold her nurturing and life-supporting energies. And just as the Earth can stifle and suffocate, an overly tenacious Mother can overwhelm and inhibit a child's natural inclination to grow and individuate.

Sympathy, the emotion of the Earth Element, contains a similar paradox. When given appropriately and without ulterior motives, sympathy can act as a balm that helps us heal and move on with the unfolding of our own entelechy. However, when engaged unconsciously or manipulatively, sympathy can become toxic. Excess sympathy blurs the boundary between my own experience and the

The Alchemy of Inner Work

experience of another. It carries with it the risk of fixation on another person's suffering and a deterioration of separateness that can pull us back into the fusional mother/child identification of infancy. Lack of sympathy is equally stunting to growth. It can be likened to gardening in a soil without nutrients and water, a garden where the fullness of growth is unsupported.

Sympathy, while an intrinsic and necessary part of the Earth Element and the Mother archetype, is potentially entropic, easily downgraded into merging, over-identification, self-pity, impasse, and stagnation. Another possibility emerges if you can access the legacy of Earth's grandparent, the Wood Element, and stay connected to your own defined plan while maintaining clear boundaries as you engage with another person's experience. Then your sympathy for another is appropriately limited and qualified. Sympathy transforms into empathy as you feel and resonate with another while always remembering that you are not them.

Instead of saying, "I know how you feel," empathy says, "I am present with you as you feel your feelings and I feel mine."

Transforming sympathy into empathy is an ongoing practice that we must re-engage on a daily basis. Remembering to come back to yourself and your own inner experience as you take in the experience of another person allows you to hold your center. Being as close as you can to another's suffering while remembering the sacredness of the distance between you allows you to make a space for the healing power of the Divine Mother, while honoring the limitations of your own humanity.

Discovering Earth Within You

Are your words and your actions in integrity with each other?
Your lead:

- You over-mother, worry, feel sorry for others or yourself, infantilize, pity, meddle, and coddle.

- You lose sight of your own edge and give at the expense of your own well-being, nourishment, and growth.

- You can't digest experiences and get stuck in perseveration and unclear thinking; you experience blockages in the form of phlegm, dampness, obsession, and repetitive cogitation.

Your gold:

- You have a clear, focused yet spacious and unattached mind and feel grounded and secure in your life.

- Your healthy physical and psychic digestion transforms nourishment into freely moving energy and empowered action.

- You balance your caring for yourself with your caring for others.

- You feel grounded and secure in your life.

The harvest of Late Summer fruit stabilizes and materializes the sunlight that has poured down on the plant world through Summer. It makes this vital energy available to other beings in the form of food. But unless this matter—the product of the Earth Season—is actively used, eaten, transformed, or digested and given back to the soil in the form of minerals, it will rot or desiccate. All that Earth produces must ultimately be sacrificed in service to the turning of the Wheel.

As the air cools and the Late Summer sun dips lower in the sky, it is time to let go and surrender the gifts of Earth to the Goddess who waits below in the darkness of the underworld. Have you received enough of Earth's bounty to surrender it all to her? Have you found a center that you can hold inside yourself when everything around you disintegrates? Are you able to get as close as you can to another while remembering yourself?

Metal: Quintessence

Autumn/Composting Plant Matter/Mineral Essences

The Metal Element is related to Autumn. During this time of the yearly cycle, as daytime diminishes and nights lengthen, vital forces contract inward, and life-giving moisture drains from the exterior leading to dormancy. Leaves shrivel and die. Seeds harden and fall to the ground. Metal expresses the introverting, sequestering wisdom of nature as it prepares to meet the challenges of Winter. Life essences must be gathered, hidden away, and kept safe.

Yet, in the most impenetrable recesses of this surrender of outward growth, at the base of the sacrifice, the descent, the drying, hardening, and decomposing, is the secret dream of Metal's child. As Autumn turns toward the long, dark nights of Winter, the faith of Water is buried in every seed, a faith so impossible that it is barely whispered: life will return and "I surrender to transformation" will again become "I am!"

Downward/Canopy-Like/Letting Go/Grief

Metal's placement at the bottom of the Wheel affirms our understanding of its energetic nature, its tendency to slow and eventually arrest the movement of growth, to draw the life force down toward what is yin, dark, cold, inward, and still. At this point on the Wheel, there is a restriction of growth, a pressure down into the depths, and a long exhalation.

Along with this exhale, this release and letting go, there is an inhalation, an impulse to gather and preserve, condense, concentrate, and sequester what is most precious and essential to life. This aspect of Metal is associated with the shape of a canopy, a covering that functions to protect as well as store. The canopy is mirrored in the physical shape of the lungs, the organ associated with the Metal Element, which hang down like a roof over the heart as well as the other organs in the lower torso.

The Emotion is Grief. Grief out of balance shows up as negativity, despair, depression, an intractable holding on to the past. However, when the influence of Metal is honored, the emotion of Grief is a release of holding, an awesome surrender in the face of the infinite. Standing steady in the face of our own limits, the lungs expand, and we can receive the inspiration of the Heavens.

Alchemy: Transforming Grief into Presence

As I walk alone through the late November twilight, I notice the air is filled with emptiness. October's multicolored patchwork of leaves is now a straggle of torn gold rattling on bare black branches. The veil between the worlds of life and death has grown thin.

Sometimes I go to the cove by my home to sit on a stone and watch the water. This stone, where my mother also sat for so many summers, is cold now. I miss my mother every day, and this missing reminds me of clouds, of something precious that is slipping through my fingers like a fine mist.

A year or so ago, I walked down to the shore and discovered that the land had been broken open, a hole had been dug, and a foundation poured. This new house is the latest of many developments in a place that has been sacred to me. At first, I did not want to go back, but I returned to watch the tide and the small brown ducks who winter here.

Metal requires that we not turn back from the darkness. It invites us to breathe deep into loss and not avert our gaze from the tragedy of our own story, our own time. Metal tells me that if I turn away from what I cannot bear, my life will be lost to me.

Often, the sadness feels like too much. Words scatter in the winds, meaning is swallowed by the void that breathes patiently on the other side of my daily life, and all I want to do is close my eyes and sleep. But by taking my time, breathing into my grief, and saying yes instead of no to the restriction and the loss, something opens in my being.

In this way, I can stay present to my circumstances. In this way, I can dare to leap into a night without dreams, without bottom, and without end. I can wait. I can listen. And I can surrender into trust that I'll begin to see in the darkness.

In a state of imbalance, the Emotion of Metal shows up as rigidity, a clinging to the past, stubborn depression, and unrelenting mourning that completely engulfs your life. It does not shift with the passage of time. In health, Grief expresses as a willingness to accept the inevitability of loss and to embrace the preciousness of each passing moment. At its best, the Grief of Metal shows as a spiritual acceptance and spaciousness that brings peace and mindful presence to everyone it touches.

Discovering Metal Within You

Are you capable of letting go, receiving inspiration, and being in a place of not knowing?

Your lead:

- You are isolated and imprisoned by rigidity and resistance to change.

- Your inability to recognize what is essential and precious leads to hoarding and over-accumulation of stuff, ideas, and emotion.

- Your inability to come to terms with the finite nature of material existence and the great teaching of death leads to a failure of spiritual maturity.

Your gold:

- You transform your desperate fear of emptiness into the spacious serenity of not knowing.

- You receive inspiration from Heaven, spirit, and the shining illumination of the divine.

- You are in touch with the preciousness of life and each passing moment.

Psychologically, Metal teaches us about the inevitability of change and loss. Along with its lessons of restraint, restriction, and ending, Metal offers liberation. As you traverse this closing phase of the cycle, you are invited to open to a larger sense of who you are. Yielding to the power of the master craftperson's hand, trusting the knowing of the star that tumbled into you at the moment of your conception, you move beyond the limitations of individual ego identity and personal will and surrender to the infinite. As you relinquish your grasp on perfection, static form, or predictable outcome, you join the sage and the crone who dance at the edges of time. In ultimately requiring you to let go of your clinging and control of life, Metal teaches you at last how to truly live.

Chapter 9

The Alchemical
Medicine Cabinet

*Each star influences its own substance, and according to their peculiar
nature, they produce different things. They work first in heaven above,
then in the earth beneath in the elements, each according to its own
peculiar virtue.*

—John Mehung, *A Demonstration of Nature*

Fuchsia

I open the old wood cabinet and sort through the rows of alphabet-
ized bottles. I am preparing a mix of flower essences for a patient. I
envision this patient in my mind's eye. I call up the feeling of being
with her, the particular way she moves through the world.

The picture is clear to me: a woman in her mid-twenties heading
off to graduate school. Androgynous and Puck-like, she is good at
making green things grow in gardens, playing chess, baking bread,
charming women as well as men. She is a balanced mix of strength
and vulnerability, coolness and warmth; she is self-assured, compe-
tent, thoughtful, and emotionally contained. In her presence, certain
images arise for me: an alert young fox in a field, a willow tree in
Spring, Artemis the Virgin Huntress, and every so often when she
tilts her head in a particular way, I see an old wise crow peeking out
from behind her still-girlish face.

She has asked for support as she moves into the next chapter of her life. She is beginning an intensive, competitive program in a big, new city. Between sentences, she pauses. She clears her throat. She mentions something about not knowing how to let people in, some feeling inside she can't exactly pin down. Then the conversation turns to knee pain, finding a part-time job, the upcoming internship. Then, another turn and she is telling me of a friend who used to be a lover who she thinks, maybe, she might want to call. And then there's another, who she also loves but isn't sure what to do with.

She pauses again and takes a breath. "Maybe it's best to let them all go," she says. Start fresh, focus on her own life, her own work. But then, she wants to stay connected, she wants to feel something. She is silent. Then she speaks again: "I don't like big emotions. And I like keeping my options open."

Remembering this exchange, I peruse the cabinet. I pick Walnut for smooth transition and clarity of identity, stability of self during times of change; Pink Yarrow for appropriate emotional boundaries, loving connections with others while maintaining awareness of personal needs, for compassion with clarity; Trumpet Vine, the impetuous and determined climber with its over-abundance of orange bell-shaped blossoms, for a clear, strong voice, ease, and elegance of expression, the ability to speak one's truth without hesitation and flowing sentences that come from the heart.

It is early August. Outside the office window, the Fire Element is peaking on the coast of Maine. There are flowers in every color. Everywhere. I am finished for the day, ready to get outside. But an internal tug pulls me back to the cabinet. Something is still missing in this mix—another flower essence wants in. I can't put my finger on the missing piece. I am feeling a bit impatient with the process, eager to get down to the cove for a swim. Still, I just don't feel the click in my body that says the mix is complete.

Then I see it hanging in the basket just outside the screen door. It's spilling over the edges of its pot, unabashedly seductive, dozens and dozens of small pink and magenta faces, lips and tongues exposed, dripping with nectar, showing off, showing up, yet looking down, ever so slightly hiding from the direct rays of the sun. Fuchsia. That's the missing piece.

But then I doubt myself. She doesn't match the classic textbook picture for Fuchsia flower essence at all. The conditions suggested for this essence are false hyper-emotionality and hysteria, multiple physical complaints masking true feelings. This patient is one of the least histrionic women I know, reliably appropriate and economical in her emotional expression. As for multiple physical complaints, she's in fine health aside from some minor knee pain after she ran a half marathon in the early Spring.

I prepare the mix with the three flowers that make rational sense. Good. Done. I am ready to close the cabinet. Once again, outside the screen door the fuchsia flowers tremble in the breeze, gorgeously, excessively adorned in their petal gowns, hats, and veils. Calling for attention, they want into the mix. But I still don't understand why.

Then I see another flash of ruby red followed by an almost intrusive mechanical buzz. A bird no bigger than my thumb. Spinning, twirling on its translucent wings, poking the finely formed curve of its narrow beak into one blossom and then another. Dipping in and out but never staying still long enough to be caught. Back and forth and back again, but always keeping its distance from the cup of abundance, the rich fiery beauty of the flowers.

It's the feeling of that tiny hummingbird with its wings beating like an anxious heart, never stopping, never staying, hovering just above the deep dip down into the blood red center of the flower. Hovering resolutely just above surrender. That's the missing piece. It's about the relationship between the bird and the flower. It's about opening up to a different level of emotional communication. It's about moving past her fear of depth.

When I give her the mix, I tell her about the flowers I chose and why. The Walnut. The Pink Yarrow. The Trumpet Flower. They all make sense. And then, I mention Fuchsia.

"It doesn't seem right," I say. "You don't fit the classic picture. I've never seen you hysterical. You aren't a hypochondriac. I don't feel that there is some hidden trauma you are running from. But this flower wanted to be included. It was literally tapping at the window as I prepared this mix. I kept sitting with it. I wondered. Maybe there are some big feelings inside that you are having a hard time expressing. Maybe you stay a little above your emotions by moving from one person to another. Maybe you are holding back, staying busy, never opening beyond a certain point. Does any of that click for you?"

She looked at me, her eyes wide. "How did you get that? After our last session, I had a total emotional meltdown. That never happens to me. I always keep my emotions under control. But I realized I'm feeling so alone right now. I want to be able to talk about what I'm feeling inside with the people I'm close to. But I'm afraid it will be too big, too dramatic. I'll be too much. So, I keep it all inside and forget about the loneliness. I don't want to do that anymore. How did you know all that was going on? I feel like you really see me. See what I need. How did you do that?"

A Different Kind of Knowing

The answer to my patient's question "How did you do that?" is both simple and complex. I didn't do it alone. I had help. To understand the answer requires that we relinquish our hold on mental consciousness—our linear, rational approach to reality. We need to trust a more fluid, multidimensional kind of knowing and we need to open to a different way of viewing the therapeutic relationship.

Alchemy has always been practiced as a nondual process, meaning that alchemists recognize both the separation and unity of all things. They regard connections, intersections, and the interweaving of experiences as equal in importance to distinctions, dissections, and analysis. They focus on the field between polarities such as subject and object, seer and seen, mind and body, matter and spirit, and are interested in the mutable flux of insights that arise rather than fixed ideas that emerge from a single perspective.

When you approach a healing process alchemically, you are attending to an "in-between" space where dualities mingle, marry, and merge in order to give birth to new possibilities. Polarities become bride and bridegroom in the domain of the soul—home to the celestial meeting of opposites. This is a domain that you cannot perceive with the ordinary senses or know through your rational mind alone. In order to see in this way, you must open your heart to another kind of seeing, hearing, and knowing.

The answer to my patient's question "How did I know?" begins with another question: "Who is the knower?"

Looking through the screen door of my alchemical laboratory, it may be the fuchsia blossoms themselves that know what my patient needs, or it may be my patient communicating what she needs to me nonverbally through the flower. Or it may be a part of me that needs to learn more about passion and its expression and my patient who is offering me the gift of this learning. From an alchemical perspective, I know what my patient needs because, although we are distinct individuals, my patient and I are also deeply connected through a substratum of knowing that pervades the field of our relationship as well as the entire cosmos. From this perspective, my patient's healing is connected to my own. My patient, the flower, and I are all agents and recipients, participating in a single divine act of healing that may also help in some small way to heal the world.

Stirring the Life Force/Touching the Soul

Anything that moves the qi can be used as a tool in Alchemical Healing. From an image to a flower essence, a crystal to an oil, a word to a needle, the distinguishing feature of an alchemical tool is that its spirit, its inner star, has been illuminated. Its archetypal dimension and its capacity to touch the human soul is activated. In this way, an ordinary stainless-steel needle transforms into a celestial pivot, the fulcrum of a patient's healing process. A small drop of rose oil becomes an elixir to heal a broken heart. A point name helps answer the riddle of a patient's depression. A dream suggests a way to resolve a seemingly impossible impasse. A few drops of water touched by the essence of Summer flowers can begin to shift an emotional pattern that has been in place for a lifetime.

The alchemical transmutation of your healing tools does not happen by chance. It does not come from studying point compendiums, charts, textbooks or webinars, although this too is important. It has nothing to do with packaging or exotic, expensive ingredients. Rather, it comes from your work with these tools in the laboratory of your own body and soul. The deeper healing capacities come to life through your devotion and personal engagement with the tools over time. It comes from your bringing multiple forms of awareness to your investigations of the point, the oil, the myth or the dream image as well as to the treatment.

In order to transform an ordinary medicinal, needle, point name, touch, story, stone, dream, or anything else that touches the qi into an alchemical tool, you invite it into your inner laboratory. You approach it as a being with a soul and an intelligence of its own. You sit next to it, befriend it, relate to it with care and consciousness. You look at it not only with your "ordinary" everyday eyes but also with the multi-dimensional eyes of your heart. Anything that moves the qi *can* be used as a tool in Alchemical Healing; and yet, alchemy doesn't just happen. It takes time, imagination, relationship, intention, humility, and faith.

You get curious about the likes and the dislikes of the Rock Rose flower. You wonder how its habitat reflects something about the flower essence's capacity to help a person recover from shock. You learn about the knife wounds on the Frankincense tree from which the oil is extracted and wonder how the scarring of the tree influences the character of the oil.

The next important step is the setting of intention. From an alchemical perspective, intention is not an abstract idea. It is an energetic force that is the cornerstone of an alchemical process. Bringing a clear intention to your use of a tool directs and potentizes its effects. In my own practice, as I pick up a tool, I consciously commit to using it to promote the arising of some new possibility in a person's life as opposed to simply helping them get back to their old self again. I feel the intention take root in my whole body. I send it through the needle and infuse it in the flower essence or oil mixes I prepare.

Staying connected to this intention helps me resist the impulse to try to prematurely fix a symptom or, conversely, to shy away from touching on a person's lead—the stuck, difficult areas where the new possibilities may be hiding. It allows me to hold steady when things get rocky in a treatment process and to act as a kind of stabilizing central axis for my patients until they are able to feel their own stability.

In addition to the above attitudes and actions, there is another quality that I believe is a crucial prerequisite for alchemical work. That is humility. While I recognize the central importance of my clearly stated intention, I also understand that my intention is a force that I must join with the spirit of the substance or tool I am working with, an "other" with its own intelligence, wisdom, and intention whose divinity I must honor if I want to unleash its healing power. In this work, the conscious ego has a role to play but it is not in charge. Transformation happens when the time is right and the Self is ready, not when our egos want it to happen. It is the crucial task of consciousness to create, and to continue to create, the conditions necessary in order for the magic of healing to arise. While I always try to bring intention, patience, care and relationship to the tools I work with, I also try to remember the human-size limitations of my own capacities. I find that the healing process works best when I can be okay with the limits of my knowing.

The Alchemical Healing Medicine Cabinet

In the following pages, I share five of my favorite flower essences and essential oils. I have chosen flower essences from the Bach line as they are easily obtained in most health food stores. I associate each one of these medicinals with a particular Element—Water, Wood, Fire, Earth, or Metal—and present these ten medicinals as a basic starter Alchemical Healing Medicine Cabinet.

If you are just beginning to work with these tools, I suggest that you start with these ten medicinals until you feel that you have an embodied sense of who they are and what they do. As you delve more deeply into this work, you will add many others; however, from an alchemical perspective it is far better to know a few medicinals deeply than to have many that you know superficially. If you work with these ten plant allies as a practice over time, you will be surprised by how far they will take you.

Be certain you purchase pharmaceutical grade oils (see the Appendix for suggestions). Although rose and frankincense are relatively expensive oils, a ¼ dram (1mL) bottle is all you need to get started. If you use these oils according to the directions given here, that little bottle will last several months to a year.

Flower Essences

Flower essences contain the vibrational or soul imprint of the plants used to create them, but almost no material residue of the plant itself. They were first developed by English bacteriologist, pathologist, and homeopath Dr. Edward Bach in the 1930s. Dr. Bach identified a repertory of thirty-eight remedies that addressed basic issues of the body, mind, and spirit. Today, there are hundreds of other essences that have been developed by practitioners around the world and you can create your own from the plants that grow in your particular environment.

Flower essences play an important role in Alchemical Healing. They are the quintessential spirit-level remedy, as most are made from flower blossoms, the part of plants most closely related to the Fire Element and to the shen. Many essences are produced by shining sunlight through the plant material as the blossoms float in a bowl of water, sequestering the activated light in a material substance.

Acupuncturist and master flower essence practitioner Lindsay Fauntleroy views flower essences as primary agents of alchemical transformation. In her words,

> The flowers, taken over time, catalyze shifts at the level of
> our souls that result in unexpected miracles in our outer lives.
> Flower essences invite us to welcome ancestral understandings
> of health, humanity, and the cosmos into a modern context. Just
> like Sankofa, the African mythological bird that flies forward
> into the future while seeing deep into the past, these ancient

ways of knowing are critical to the success of an emerging healing paradigm that honors the mind, body and soul connection.

Flower essences are gentle yet powerful allies at every stage of a healing process. They are safe for people of any age and level of health or illness. They are nontoxic, have no side effects, are not habit forming, and do not interfere with other medications, pharmaceutical or herbal. There are many ways you can use flower essences and only a few specific stipulations you should observe when considering them. Flower essences can also be used as a powerful intervention in emergency situations. They are equally effective as a support in transforming long entrenched psychological patterns and character traits as well as passing moods and temporary emotional challenges.

Flower Essences Directions for Use

For emergencies and passing moods, add 2 drops of each chosen remedy to a small glass of water. Sip at intervals throughout the day until emotions settle.

For addressing long-standing issues, fill a 30 mL (1 oz.) sterilized glass dropper bottle with spring or filtered water, the most pristine source available. Add 5–10 drops of your chosen essences (with a maximum of six essences). Add 1 tablespoon of brandy or vodka as a preservative. Take the blend under the tongue at least four times a day, 4 drops each time, for a minimum of twenty-eight days before reassessing. Changes are likely to be subtle or surprisingly unexpected. Sometimes, you barely notice that anything happens until some weeks later you realize you forgot all about the problem or issue you identified to work on.

Flower essences can be applied full strength to specific acupuncture points or diluted 2–4 drops in 4–6 oz. of water and applied with a cotton ball to an entire meridian. Apply the essence to the point and rest for ten minutes. The essence and point will join vibrations and initiate change. See the next chapter for point prescriptions and protocols.

Due to the sensitive nature of flower essences, don't let the glass applicator of the dropper bottle touch your skin or tongue. If it does, dip the applicator in alcohol to clean it. If you are alcohol sensitive, you can drop the essences in a bit of boiling water to evaporate the alcohol before swallowing. There are also essences that are preserved in glycerin rather than alcohol. See the Appendix for sources. Negative treatment responses are rare. In general, when the remedy is not right for the person, there is little or no response to the treatment. If there is no change after twenty-eight days, discontinue use and explore another flower essence or blend.

Five Alchemical Flower Essences

Water: Rock Rose

Nature: Rock Rose is a low-growing shrub found throughout most of Europe that thrives in dry, poorly nourished soil. As its Latin name, *Helianthemum nummuralium*, suggests, this is a sun-loving flower that produces vivid flowers in shades of orange, pink, yellow, and white in the late Spring to early Summer months.

Alchemy: One of the key alchemical traits of this flower is found in its seeds, which remain dormant for long periods of time buried deep in the soil. This dormancy capacity allows the seeds to survive drought and wildfire and to renew quickly after landscape devastation.

Use: Rock Rose is the quintessential healer when the Water Element is undernourished, stressed, or undermined by trauma, resulting in fear, shakiness, and deep emotional upset. It supports recovery from acute shock as well as from chronic states of anxiety and panic. Rock Rose brings courage and resiliency as well as composure and presence of mind. It is the flower to turn to for survival and recovery during and after challenging times.

Wood: Gorse

Nature: Like Rock Rose, Gorse thrives in difficult conditions and is often found growing alone in dry, rocky soil. It is a thorny evergreen shrub with yellow flowers that blossom profusely in Spring.

Alchemy: As a member of the pea family, one of this plant's key alchemical traits is its ability to fix nitrogen from the air. The nitrogen then infiltrates the soil and helps other plants of the same species establish themselves despite the sparse nutrient condition of the soil.

Use: Gorse is the healer to call on when the growth capacities and forward direction of the Wood Element are blocked and impaired. It transforms feelings of repressed anger—resignation, bitterness, and reactivity—into a healthy aggression and hope for the future that allows you to thrive in the face of adversity and go for what you want. Gorse transforms negativity and self-protectiveness into a sunny optimism and generosity that nourishes, heals, and brings others closer rather than pushing them away.

Fire: Holly

Nature: Holly is an evergreen tree with green glossy sharp-thorned leaves and shimmering red Winter berries. It is one of the only evergreen trees native to the British Isles. For this reason, the Celts associated it with the returning light of the Winter solstice season. With the advent of Christianity, it became known as Christmas holly.

Alchemy: Holly berries are protected by the thorny leaves but also by their late Winter ripening, which allows them to adhere strongly to their branches during the first months of cold weather. After the solstice chill, the berries soften, drop to the ground, and become an important source of food for birds when few other sources are available. Holly's alchemy lies in its ability to protect yet at the same time appropriately share the beauty and nourishment of its crimson fruit.

Use: Turn to Holly when the Fire Element has been wounded by a disappointment in love, a painful betrayal, or abandonment, resulting in defensive armoring. When there is excessive protection (spikes) around the crimson flame of the heart, Holly gently opens its portals so that the spirit can shine through without dismantling the capacity for discernment and healthy boundaries. Jealousy, suspicion, and isolation transform into compassion, gratitude, and an openness to connection, friendship, and love.

Earth: Centaury

Nature: Centaury is a tough plant that grows on chalky cliffs and in dry pastures. It is an extremely bitter plant that seems to have a fine sense of its own preferences. It loves the sun and its flowers open only in fine weather and not after mid-day.

Alchemy: This plant is named for the Centaurs, the mythical half-human, half-horse creatures who appeared in mythology from the time of the early Greeks. Centaurs symbolize the liminal world between animal and human and hold the tension between instinct and wisdom. One of the most famous Centaurs, Chiron, is renowned for his knowledge, kindness, healing, and teaching abilities. In one version of the Chiron myth, he cured himself from a wound inflicted by an arrow poisoned by the blood of the strangling monster Hydra. Thus, Centaury was an important remedy in ancient Greece, where it was used to heal infected wounds. Later, Saxon herbalists prescribed it to restore the life force after snake bites and other poisonous infections.

Use: I turn to Centaury when the ego forces are weak and a person is taken over, "strangled" by the needs of others. In other words, when the Earth Element has lost its capacity to know what it needs and devotes itself exclusively to the needs of others at the expense of its own well-being and growth. Centaury helps you get in touch with your own inner wisdom and individual truth free from outside influences. It endows you with the inner strength to say no when necessary along with the healing wisdom that allows you to help others when appropriate.

Metal: Rock Water

Nature: This essence is the only one of the thirty-eight Bach flower essences that is not made from a flower, but rather from a dilution of spring water that has percolated up between stones deep in the earth and then solarized with sunlight.

Alchemy: Spring water gradually wears away and reforms the hard, calcified stone that it makes contact with. It also has the capacity to receive and be transformed by the warmth and energy of the sun.

Use: Consider Rock Water when the Metal Element has become cold, brittle, and lifeless. This is the essence of choice when a person's creativity and enjoyment of life are diminished by rigid attitudes, restrictive discipline, and unrealistic ideals. This sense of restraint can take the form of extreme and strict dieting, grueling exercise routines, inflexible schedules, uncompromising religious dogma, and judgmental attitudes. Just as spring water gradually softens and reshapes stone, Rock Water moderates and reforms overly crystallized habits and self-imposed limiting structures. It is a powerful remedy for people who need to develop more flexibility and ease or joy in life.

Essential Oils

The distillation of essential oils from aromatic plants has been an important part of alchemical practice for centuries. The complex technology of distillation was developed sometime in the sixth century, most likely by Persian alchemists. Later the technology spread to Europe and India. Distillation of herbs, flowers, and aromatic woods began in China around the same time and may have come to China from the Middle East.

Correctly used, essential oils offer a safe, effective, and fast-acting way to work on many levels. They calm the emotions and shift states of mind. They help regulate sleep and dreaming but also support focus, alertness, and energy. They support clarity of thought and strong intention. Over time, use of essential oils can help clear toxins on both physical and emotional levels, support immunity, and relax the autonomic nervous system. At the deepest levels of our being, essential oils calm and strengthen the adrenals, and strengthen the sense of self and well-being.

From a physiological perspective, fragrance—the therapeutically active aspect of the oil—bypasses the digestive organs and tissues and enters through the respiratory system and olfactory senses. As smell is processed by ancient parts of our nervous system that have to do with survival, the brain registers aroma twice as fast as it does pain. This is why inhalation can powerfully and almost immediately transform the emotions.

Although essential oils, when correctly administered, are non-toxic, safe, and have relatively few negative side effects, they must be used with care. Essential oils are powerful, fast-acting medicinals with strong personalities that call for respect and wisdom.

There are three basic safety guidelines for using essential oils. The first is not to take essential oils internally unless you have advanced training in pharmacology and medicine. The second is not to apply essential oils directly to skin without diluting them in a carrier oil, except in the case of using a pinhead-size drop on an acupuncture point. You can check for skin sensitivity by applying an oil to a very small area of skin. The last safety guideline is to not use essential oils during pregnancy or post-partum unless you have advanced training.

In addition, if you are taking pharmaceutical drugs, monitor your response to the introduction of essential oils. You may need to discuss with you doctor an adjustment of dosage when you introduce the oils. Specifically, if you are on a blood thinner medication, only use essential oils if your doctor is monitoring "clotting time." Always stay aware of your body and listen to its response. Everyone metabolizes oils differently. If you experience increased urination after using oils for some time, you may want to consider reducing your use.

Here are a number of ways to work safely with essential oils:

Direct palm inhalation. Sprinkle a few drops of diluted oil on the palms, rub your hands together, and inhale.

Massage and body oils. The best carriers are coconut, jojoba, and sesame oil, although you will again want to make sure you are not sensitive to any of these carriers by rubbing a small amount on your skin. Dilute the essential oil in the carrier a few drops at a time until you achieve the level of fragrance you desire. Use this scented oil to massage the back of your neck and shoulders or anywhere on your body for relaxation and stress relief.

Bath. Do not drop essential oils directly into bath water, where it will collect in droplets and possibly irritate your skin. Instead, put a few drops of oil in milk, honey, or salt to emulsify it. Add the emulsified oil to your bath as the tub fills. The dose used for aromatic baths is very low, in the range of 5 to 10 drops, depending on the oil.

Aromatherapy. Add 5 to 10 drops of oil to a half ounce of carrier oil and apply it to specific points or inhale the oil as needed.

Steam inhalation. Add 2 to 4 drops of essential oil to a basin of hot water. Form a tent with a towel over your head and inhale. Be careful that the steam does not burn your eyes.

When choosing a carrier oil to use with essential oils, consider the qualities associated with these popularly used oils:

- Jojoba oil is hypo-allergenic and suitable for most mixes.

- Safflower oil invigorates the blood and is a moving oil to use in abdominal rubs when there is stagnation.

- Sweet almond oil is gentle and moistening to the skin.

- Sesame oil warms, sedates, and gently tonifies. It is nice massaged into the soles of the feet at night; cover with cotton socks to relax and induce a good night's sleep.

- Peach kernel oil is neutral.

- Coconut oil is particularly good for massaging tight muscles.

Five Alchemical Essential Oils

Water: Balsam Fir

Nature: Balsam fir thrives in cool climates and moist soil. It is known for its unique aroma that is especially potent after the tree is wounded or cut.

Alchemy: The word *balsam* is used in alchemy to refer to a substance—a balm—that has deep, even sacred, healing properties. In the early laboratories, this balm was produced by a process of distillation of red sulfur and white lime that resulted in a dark reddish-brown essence considered an exudation of the soul. The sticky brownish-golden sap of the fir is the "balm" this oil is made from.

Use: I use Balsam Fir essential oil when the Water Element calls for its deeply calming, rooting, and at the same time wildly invigorating fragrance. You can apply it topically in diluted form to ease discomfort in aching joints and muscles. Additionally, it has antimicrobial properties, so rub a few drops on your palm and inhale if you are exposed to Winter coughs and colds. A student and colleague described her understanding of this oil beautifully: "It is the essence of evergreen and what is evergreen within us. The scent instills hope, brings a feeling of expansion punctuated by consolidation . . . it is my go-to oil for seasonal depressive disorder . . . it brings the smell of Winter's light, even if the sun is hidden by clouds and is physically further away from us by the tilt of our axis."

Wood: Bergamot

Nature: Bergamot is a citrus tree that bears a fruit in mid-Winter about the size of a small orange. The oil is made from the green peel of the unripe fruit.

Alchemy: The spirit of this fruit is such a potent qi mover and spirit lifter that even just thinking about it will cause your taste buds to tingle and your salivary glands to produce fluids once you are familiar with its scent. Imagine a few drops of lemon juice on your tongue and you've got it. Chinese herbalists have understood this property for centuries and have incorporated citrus peel as an important ingredient in the herbal treatment of stuck qi, depression, impaired digestion, and stagnation.

Use: Relaxing and at the same time uplifting, Bergamot releases and harmonizes stagnant liver qi and supports the uninhibited flow of the Wood Element. As a result of its qi moving properties, it brings suppressed emotions to the surface, liberates the healthy

The Alchemy of Inner Work

aggression trapped in depression, and transforms pent-up frustration into free-flowing hope. I mix Bergamot essential oil with a carrier oil and massage it into the area just below the ribs, especially over the liver area on the right side and mid-thoracic area of the back. Like all citrus oils, Bergamot oil can increase sensitivity to light, so avoid exposure to the sun after application of this oil to the skin.

Fire: Rose

Nature: There are at least 350 known rose species and more than 10,000 hybrid varieties but it is the single species, *Rosa damascena* or damask rose, cultivated since the sixteenth century, that is most prized for medicinal essential oil. It takes up to 60,000 roses to produce one small bottle of oil.

Alchemy: Like Holly, the rose protects its exquisite and delicate blossom with sharp prickles and thorns. According to alchemist and author Dennis William Hauck, no flower inspired European alchemists more. He writes,

> The rose is more meaningful, much older, and more deeply embedded in the human subconscious than most people believe . . . it is a paradoxical symbol of both purity and passion, heavenly perfection and earthy desire, life and death . . . a symbol of joy . . . as well as secrecy and silence . . . and romantic love.

Use: Rose is the most important essential oil for the heart and the Fire Element. When you use this oil, you tap into the wisdom of the plant in its fullest expression of creativity, blossoming, and trust. Rose oil is a cool, moist essence that provides gentle support and protection for the soul. It opens the heart to love while at the same time augmenting the capacity for appropriate caution. It alleviates depression and restores a sense of wellbeing and joy. It is particularly useful in addressing emotional wounds from loss, rejection, and betrayal, and allows you to be present to what is rather than struggling to recover what is not. Symptomatically, this oil alleviates anxiety, induces restful sleep, and promotes creative dreaming. The one caveat for Rose oil is that it is crucial to find a good quality, completely natural oil. Doing so can be quite expensive; however, a little bit goes a long way and a few drops in a carrier oil are sufficient for most uses.

Earth: Coriander

Nature: Coriander, also known as cilantro, is a widely distributed annual herb. It has a spicy, perky, enlivening energy that captures the flavor and aroma of high Summer.

Alchemy: For me, coriander has a penetrating specificity, an aroma and flavor completely unlike any other. Interestingly, these qualities are completely different from its "mother plant," cilantro. This specificity reflects for me a capacity to differentiate itself from its matrix, to produce something new out of its own being.

Use: This oil supports the Earth Element by clearing phlegm, aiding digestion, and supporting clarity of the mind. Coriander roots and stabilizes while at the same time imbuing a feeling of liveliness and spontaneity. A student and colleague described coriander this way:

> It was like an immediate lift-off from the back of my nose, behind my eyes, up to my scalp and spine. I felt immediate energy and a prickling kind of jazzy, pointed, floating ascendance. I'm calling it the spicy lemon-green expansion. I feel like I could go out and run a marathon or shake a hundred people's hands. The image that comes to me is being in a musty, closed up hut deep in the forest and throwing open the door to the green outdoors!

Metal: Frankincense

Nature: Frankincense is one of the oldest known fragrant oils. It is derived from the Boswellia tree, which is native to North Africa and the Middle East.

Alchemy: Frankincense essential oil is made from the milky aromatic resin, sometimes called "tears," extracted from wounds intentionally cut into the bark of the tree. The resin has been traded for use as a sacred aromatic incense for more than 6,000 years. Together with the incense myrrh, it is said to be one of the gifts brought by the Magi to celebrate the birth of Christ. The fact that this oil comes from wounds in the tree's bark tells you something about its capacity to heal deep emotional and spiritual scars. It allows you to experience the sacredness of loss and to open yourself to the support of energies that come from beyond your own limited conscious awareness.

Use: This is an oil with profound spiritual wisdom that supports the Metal Element in receiving the inspiration of the divine. The oil supports deep introspection, meditation, and prayer while safe guarding us from negative thoughts and influences. It is known for its capacity to heal wounds and scars on the skin and I have found it to have profound effects in healing wounds and scars at the level of the soul and the spirit as well.

Chapter 10

Points and Portals

> ... [I]f one pays close attention ... shen, the spirit, becomes clear to
> man as though the wind has blown away the cloud.
>
> —*The Yellow Emperor's Classic of Internal Medicine,*
> trans. Ilza Veith

A Doorway Opens

The phone rings. I pick it up and it's Michael. After studying in our
mentorship program for three years while attending acupuncture
school, he graduated and launched a fast-growing Alchemical Healing and acupuncture practice in Manhattan. "Hey Michael," I say.
"What's up?"

At first, all I hear on the other end of the line is laughter. And
then in his deep former opera singer contralto, I hear him say,

> I'm getting it . . . (Pause.) . . . after all these years . . . (Pause.
> Breath.) . . . it's real. I'm understanding what you've been talking
> about. It's been happening more and more. I put the needle in a
> point and it's like a powerful wave is released. Even my patients
> are like "Whoa, what just happened?" It's as if a door opens. And
> everything shifts.

I smile and nod out the window to no one in particular. This is the moment I love, when trying to explain it is over. When it stops being an idea and becomes a Body Felt Sense knowing, when there is no longer any doubt. That you can put a tiny needle in an invisible point on the skin and watch as a person's subtle body radically transforms. He continues:

> It's amazing. Regular people, body builders and dancers, accountants and lawyers, people coming in for sprained ankles, headaches, or tight shoulders who have never heard of archetypes or alchemy or inner sensing or any of the stuff we talk about. They say, "Wow, I've had acupuncture, but this is something else!" They are feeling it. Emotions. Energy. Moving. Sensations they don't have names for. Their bodies talking, coming back to life.

"Yes, this is what keeps me in after all these years," I tell Michael. It's why I never want to quit. That feeling . . . like surfing, when I get it just right and ride in on that wave of qi . . . in that one brief moment, the whole world changes."

It can't be forced. You're never certain the magic will happen. It takes faith and devotion and it comes as a kind of grace. But Michael has experienced something that ancient Taoist alchemists knew millennia ago. Just as spirit is alive, here and now, in every particle of the cosmos, on a microcosmic level an infinitesimal speck of spirit is also present at the center of every acupuncture point. Spirit is the potent spark that ignites the movement of the qi when the point is alchemically quickened with a needle, an oil, a flower essence, an image, or a word. When you open the eyes of your heart and activate your alchemical imagination, sometimes the divine alights like a butterfly on the waiting tip of your finger.

Anything That Stirs the Qi

Michael is a trained acupuncturist who has dedicated his life to learning to stir the qi, release energy blocks, and support his patients in discovering their own Tao, but you too can learn to move the life force through the body, mind, and spirit using the simple, self-regulating strategies described in these pages. The palette of points presented in this chapter, along with the archetypes, flower essences, essential oils, and other practices presented in this book, is meant to help you open the door to your own inner alchemical laboratory and develop a relationship to your subtle body that can support you in living and feeling differently. Call on these points when you need an ally in challenging or exciting times, for emotional first aid, or to transform a piece of prima materia. This introductory alchemical point palette is not meant to be a replacement for Western medical treatment or treatment by a licensed professional acupuncturist with years of advanced training, but it will support you in engaging with your care more effectively. As you learn to work with your own qi, you improve your overall health and will indirectly support the optimal functional integration of your body, soul, and spirit. And if you continue to explore the points and meridians and open your eyes and your heart to the subtle body, you will one day feel the qi and ride in on that ephemeral wave.

The Spirit of the Point

Every acupuncture point on the body is associated with a meridian or channel of energy that runs along specific tendons and muscles and through a particular physical organ. In contemporary styles of acupuncture, each point is numbered and categorized. Each point is connected to clearly defined sets of physical symptoms and energetic imbalances.

In addition to its meridian and number, each point has a name that has been passed down over thousands of years. In many modern Chinese medical colleges these ancient names are not emphasized; however, for an Alchemical Healer the characters and imagery that make up the point name offer invaluable information. Each name carries psychological insight, spiritual wisdom, and critical clues about the usefulness of the point. For me, spending time in meditation on these names is like sitting beside a sage, a mentor who has come to me directly from the mists of time to share secrets about the inner alchemical nature of the point.

Following in the footsteps of my early teacher J. R. Worsley, I refer to the complex of imagery and meaning expressed in the point name as "the spirit of the point." When I choose to include the spirit of the point in planning a treatment, I make the wisdom and beauty contained in the name a part of the treatment process. Names such as Cloud Gate, Kunlun Mountain, Bubbling Spring, and Dove Tail have symbolic and archetypal potency. Their poetry endows sacredness to a symptom. Effectiveness then relies not only on the accurate placement of the needle but also the accurate placement of the word.

The points can attune us to the energies of the Seasons and Elements. They call our souls back to our bodies. They open us to our own potential growth. They shift the way we feel on physical and emotional levels. By relating to the points with the proper attitude and vision, they transform resentment into forgiveness, scarcity thinking into gratitude, hyper-control into acceptance. In order to bring this kind of potency to the points, you must care deeply about them. You need to re-envision your connection to them and touch them with reverence.

This chapter is not meant to be a cookbook or a how-to manual but something more akin to a letter of introduction to beloved and trusted friends. I have chosen to introduce points that sing to me and that I have come to know intimately during many years of practice. You do not have to be a trained acupuncturist to explore this simple palette of fourteen points. It takes many years of training and self-cultivation to use acupuncture needles skillfully and safely to work with complex physical and psycho-emotional symptoms, but if you bring an open heart, clear intention, and enlivened sight to your encounter with a point, it will respond to your touch and caring. If you stick with this exploration, you will gradually develop an embodied connection to the qi and facilitate positive shifts at the soul level in yourself and others you care about.

Engaging the Spirit of the Point

No one really knows how many acupuncture points there are on a human body. Some sources say 365. Some say 2,000. I say we'll never really know, and it doesn't really matter. The human body is a microcosmic reflection of the vast cosmos. Along with the mapped meridians and recognized acupuncture points, mysterious point portals appear and disappear like stars in the infinite galaxies. From the perspective of Alchemical Healing, it is not the number of points you can identify that matters, but the quality of your relationship to the points you work with. What is important is that you develop a set of points that you get to know personally, that you relate to as reliable allies.

The following entry-level point palette will allow you to begin your alchemical lab work with the points and portals of Chinese medicine. I present two points for each of the Five Elements (with an extra two for Fire), one associated with the Conception Vessel channel (the sea of yin) and one associated with the Governing Vessel channel (the sea of yang). All these points are bilateral—identically located on both sides of your body—except the Conception and Governing Vessel points, which are located on a single line that runs up the front center (Conception) and spine (Governing) of your body.

At the end of this chapter, there is a Spirit Point Map that shows the location of all fourteen points on the body. I also offer five basic protocols that include spirit points and medicinals that you can use to work alchemically with your prima materia as well as other issues in your life. I have carefully curated these points and developed these protocols for their capacity to touch the soul and to address some of the most common psycho-emotional issues I encounter in my own practice.

Spend time with these points until you feel that you have an embodied sense of who they are and what they do. Activate them with attention, imagination, touch or pressure, a flower essence, or an oil. Work with the protocols so that you can get to know the points from within your own being. I often tell my students to spend an entire Season getting deeply acquainted with just one or two points. If you work with these fourteen points as a practice over time, you will be surprised by how far they will take you!

Before You Begin

The points are organized by Element and each Element is associated with two anatomical organs or, as they are called in Chinese medicine, two Officials. Each Official is named for an organ (for example, the two Wood Element Officials are named Liver and Gallbladder). However, in Chinese medicine and Taoist alchemy, the Officials do not express physical function in the same way that they do in Western medicine. For the ancient Chinese, the organs were not simply fleshy physical structures, but rather domains of alchemical process where psychic energies—instincts, emotions, and thoughts—are tended, regulated, and transformed.

Each Official has a specific area of jurisdiction in your inner kingdom and is responsible for carrying out the soul concerns of its corresponding Element. Wood regulates the energy of sprouting and growth in you—your healthy aggression, determination, vision, and planning. When your Wood is blocked, you may feel angry, irritable, frustrated, or depressed. The Wood's two Officials, the Liver and Gall Bladder, are charged with making sure your Wood's capacity for sprouting, visioning, and planning are carried out effectively so that you can feel at ease, directed, and hopeful rather than frustrated, blocked, and hopeless as you move forward along the path of your life.

As you get acquainted with the Officials and their associated points, you may discover one or more that stand out and feel particularly relevant to your prima materia. By all means, work with the Officials that call to you but remember that an Official is not the same as an anatomical organ in the Western sense. A weakness, vulnerability, or hyperactivity of function of an Official at the alchemical level does not imply that there is pathology in your physical organ, and it is definitely not a Western medical diagnosis.

Water

The Water Officials—the Bladder and Kidney—work together to ensure you have the resources you need to become the person you are meant to be.

Your Bladder Official is in charge of regulating your fluids and energy reserves. It is responsible for the quality of your *jing*—the life essences you inherit from your parents, grandparents, and all your ancestors, the genetic memory passed from one generation to the next. The Bladder's appropriate preservation and quality control of your fluids and essences allows you to make good use of the resources you were born with as well as those that you cultivate throughout the course of your life.

Bladder 60: Kunlun Mountain

Kunlun Mountain is located on the outside of your leg in a depression just behind your ankle joint.

This point is named for the mythical mountain that was the center pole of the world, the axis of the Taoist cosmos. From high in the sky, Polaris, the North Star, pours its radiance down on Kunlun's peak where the peach tree of immortality blooms. Deep below in the mountain's labyrinths and caves, the yellow springs of life, death, and resurrection shoot upward from the dark depths. Ancient Taoist alchemists viewed Kunlun Mountain as the connecting link between Above and Below and a symbol for the Self, stabilized by the Earth and illuminated by the Heavens.

I call on this point when I feel a person's emotional spine is weak, when they don't have the resources to stand up for their own needs, or lack courage and confidence when starting a new chapter of life (leaving a marriage, beginning a new job, becoming a parent). This point also has the special ability to drain heat and overactivity from your head down through your feet. It can help when your mind is racing, your head is achy, or your shoulders and neck feel tight. Place a drop of Balsam Fir essential oil on this point, take a deep breath and receive the medicine of the tall, straight evergreens whose top-most branches scratch the stars and whose roots reach down to the reservoirs of life in the aquifers and streams of the underworld. When you need the support of Water to nourish, stabilize, and root your soul, bend down to touch this point and imagine the mountain in you rising toward the sky.

Your Kidney Official is responsible for filtering toxins and impurities in your body and making sure that clear, vital water gets to every part of your being. In addition, your Kidney Official is responsible for the storage of your jing. Through the storage, protection, and appropriate dispersal of jing, the Kidney Official safeguards your life force and helps you to live in accordance with your authentic destiny.

Kidney 1: Bubbling Spring

Bubbling Spring lives in a depression between your second and third toe on the sole of your foot.

Bubbling Spring is a center of energy for your entire body. It is the place where your feet stand, where every journey of your life begins. It is the point where the earth's revitalizing energies spring joyously up to replenish your soul. Imagine the power of sunlight melting a crack in the late Winter ice and then clear luminous spring water bubbling up from below and you will get a feeling for what this point can do.

I go to this point when a person is feeling ungrounded and hyperactivated or, conversely, dehydrated, drained, or exhausted. It is also a point I consider when someone is trying to move forward but is tentative about their own emergence.

When you touch Bubbling Spring, you tap into a powerful renewing stream of Water wisdom that will root your spirit and invigorate your entire being. This is a point of origin, a point of courage, that can connect you to the wisdom and power of your ancestry. As you touch this point, imagine you are opening to a vast river of life force, an entelechy that has flowed through your lineage and is now flowing into you from the eons of time.

Wood

The Wood Officials bring your vision into manifestation. The Liver Official is like the architect and the Gallbladder Official the head carpenter who work together to build a house.

Your Gallbladder Official is the site foreman in charge of reading the blueprint and executing the plan of your life. Choice is a key function of this Official who makes decisions and knows what direction to take next. It makes sure you have the tools, schedule, and skills you need to make your visions and plans real. Just as the twigs and branches weave the overall shape of a tree, your Gallbladder twists and turns the threads that come together to form the shape of your biography.

Gallbladder 13: Root of the Spirit

Root of the Spirit is just above your hair line directly above the outer canthus (edge) of the eye.

In late Winter, the antlers of the deer push upward, gathering the wisdom of the dark night and making way for the aggressive movements of Spring. Root of the Spirit is your "antler point." It allows you to know which way the wind is blowing and to judiciously decide when to move forward and when to rest. Root of the Spirit helps you choose the way to turn at each fork of the forest path as you move forward on your life journey.

This point can be used to relieve tension-related physical symptoms such as headache, visual dizziness, and neck tightness but these physical-level expressions represent only the most superficial aspects of the point's full nature. As its name implies, this point is a place where the spirit settles down into the body. It can be used any time you feel that your spirit has become uprooted—when you are destabilized by shock or unreasonable attacks of jealousy, worry, or confusion. As your spirit roots, you can more easily access your courage and capacity to persevere in the face of challenges. For this reason, Root of the Spirit is a very useful point for children in your life who are timid or frightened at the prospect of starting something new. This point is responsive to gentle touch and especially appreciates the application of a drop of Bergamot essential oil to relieve head tightness and open spiritual vision.

Your Liver Official is like an architect or expert military leader, constantly assessing circumstances and making plans accordingly. Your

Liver carries the vision, initiates the projects, and leads you into the creation of your future. It designs the overall shape of your tree, the blueprint, and the big overarching plan that allows you to bring the products of your imagination into form.

Liver 14: Gate of Hope

Gate of Hope is just below the bottom edge of your rib cage about two inches from the mid-line.

Where I live in Downeast Maine, just when you think it might never happen, Spring returns. The first courageous plants shoot up from the wet ground and soon the smell of green fills the air. As the Gate of Hope opens, your diaphragm relaxes and you take a deep breath as a sense of possibility returns.

On a physical level, stimulating the Gate of Hope relieves tightness in the diaphragm and the chest. On an emotional level, it relieves feelings of tension, irritability, and resentment. On a spirit level, it invites you to imagine a positive future. I like to apply a few drops of Gorse flower essence directly to this point when a person is feeling stuck, resigned, or hopeless. I will never forget the time I opened the Gate on a patient who had no knowledge of the point name and was facing the reality of her husband's alcoholism, overwhelmed with the uncertainty of whether to leave or stay in the marriage. After I needled the point, her body relaxed, she smiled, and said, "There is hope after all."

As you work with this point, visualize repressed anger transforming into healthy aggression, procrastinating fantasy into activated imagination, and acquiescence into the capacity to face adversity as you move forward into the adventure of your life.

Fire

The Fire Officials—Triple Heater, Heart Protector/Pericardium, Small Intestine, and Heart—regulate the warmth and intimacy of your relationships. They allow you to connect to yourself and to others in safe yet enlivening ways. All relationship issues are in some way connected to one of these four Officials. If you imagine the heart as a monarch seated on a throne at the center of your being, the other three Fire Officials are like the ministers charged with protecting and maintaining the heart's well-being.

Your Triple Heater Official is not related to an actual physical organ but is connected to the entire regulation of warmth in your body. The Triple Heater also helps you regulate your emotional fire as you connect to yourself and to others.

Triple Heater 6: Outer Frontier Gate

Outer Frontier Gate is on the back of your arm, in a depression between the two arm bones, about two inches from your wrist.

Imagine a great moat surrounding and protecting the kingdom of your body, mind, and spirit. At the doorway to your castle, there is a wide oak drawbridge that you can lift for privacy and safety or lower when you are ready to welcome in the resources and energies of the outside world. The Outer Frontier Gate is your energetic drawbridge. It allows you to regulate how much warmth and life force you extend to the world and how much you take it. When this drawbridge is functioning, you feel that the heat of your relationships is well-regulated, that you are receiving what you need in order to replenish what you are giving to others.

This point functions as the doorway of communication between your innermost being and the outer world. On a physical level, this is a point to turn to at the first sneeze when you feel your castle may have been "invaded" by a cold. It can help release a tight shoulder or a stiff neck so that you can more easily reach out to the world. On an emotional level, Outer Frontier Gate can help you know when you need the company of other people and when you need to be alone. It helps you assess what you actually need with regard to closeness and distance in relationships. On a spirit level, a drop of Holly flower essence on this point reminds you that you have what you need to protect yourself and that you do not have to enter an uncertain or challenging relationship encounter with the door to your heart wide open.

Your Heart Protector Official is related to the pericardium, the protective layer of tissue that envelops and protects the heart and acts as the Heart Monarch's guardian. Presiding on a more internal level than the Triple Heater, this Official's job is to act as a semi-permeable membrane that opens the way for love, warmth, and other energies that support and vitalize your heart. In health, it also effortlessly closes when negative energies approach. The smooth boundary regulation of your Heart Protector allows you to feel a sense of trust and openness to others and to yourself.

Pericardium 8: Palace of Weariness

Palace of Weariness is between your second and third finger in a depression at the center of your palm. Make a loose fist and the point will be on your palm where the tip of your middle finger lands.

At the high point of Summer, a crimson poppy bursts from its green bud and brings to fullness the promise of its minute black seed. In Chinese Medicine, this is the medicine of Fire—the capacity of the yang to expand, to open, and to move us outward into life. And yet, in order to fulfill its promise, the seed, like our own hearts, needs the protection of the bud. I envision the Palace of Weariness as the bud of the heart or as a ruby-colored dome of protection around the soul. It is also a place of convalescence where you can heal after betrayal, exhaustion, or loss, a place of preparation where you can gather your energies before moving out into the world.

This point's wisdom forms a protective, semi-permeable membrane, a shield around the heart that allows positive energies and love to enter the chamber of the Heart while effortlessly deflecting toxic or negative influences. This is a point I turn to often when a person is raw after an argument with a family member or feeling threatened in the face of a difficult meeting at work. I often use this point at the end of an initial session when a patient may feel vulnerable after speaking at length about his or her life story.

You can turn to the Palace when beginning or ending a relationship or when you want to go deeper but are feeling afraid. Of all the points in the body, this is the one that I have found most supports the paradoxical human desire to open to Self and others simultaneously.

The Small Intestine Official discerns the energies and relationships that nourish and support your heart and filters out what does not belong in your life at any given time. Like a private secretary who appraises every piece of correspondence to determine if it is worthy of the heart's attention, the Small Intestine must be able to sift through the cacophony of impressions to discern what input will actually support you in being you. The healthy Small Intestine Official listens carefully, culling out what is truly necessary, the pure from the impure, and then letting go of what doesn't serve.

Small Intestine 19: Listening Palace

Listening Palace is located in front of the tragus (the little flap that covers the front of your ear). Open your mouth a bit, press gently, and you will feel the little depression where this point lives.

Listening Palace is the point I rely on when someone has forgotten how to hear the music of their own heart. Touching this point is like bringing a small shell to your ear and hearing the sound of the ocean. It opens us to the virtue of deep listening, the capacity to discern what we truly feel and need.

I use this point when a patient is overwhelmed with input from other people and having difficulty sorting out what is truly good, nourishing, and necessary for their own heart. It is also my point of choice when a patient is having a hard time finding empathy— feeling into another person's experience without losing touch with their own truth. When you need to hear the message beyond another person's words or clarify your own heart's desires, open the door to the Listening Palace and wait in silence.

Your Heart Official is the monarch of the kingdom of your body, mind, and spirit. It is the sovereign ruler who maintains the rhythm and integrity of every other organ and activity in your body. In addition, your Heart Official is responsible for regulating the shen. It is the Official in charge of sustaining your conscious connection to your divine purpose and mandate.

Heart 7: Spirit Gate

Spirit Gate is located on the outer edge of your wrist crease at the edge of a little bone. Run your finger down a line from your pinky to your wrist and you will find this point.

At the moment of human fertilization, when the father's sperm meets the mother's egg, there is a spark that modern science now has the technology to detect. Taoist alchemists knew about this flash of fire at the moment of conception and they called it the "arrival of the spirit." From a Taoist perspective, this light organizes the development of the embryo. Eventually, it settles in the heart and directs the path of your life until the moment of your death. However, during times of upset, crisis, or emotional excitement, the shen, like a frightened bird, may fly off back to the stars from where it came. Spirit Gate opens the way for the light's return.

This point is the doorway to the innermost chamber of your heart. I call on it when trauma of any kind results in a spirit disturbance that leads to confusion or dissociation. Consider this point when your shen is agitated, when your sleep is erratic, or when you are awakened by strange dreams. When you feel anxious, disoriented, or restless, or even overly excited by joy, a drop of rose essential oil on this point will calm your shen and call the scattered birds of your spirit back to the nest of your heart.

Earth

Your Earth Officials—the Stomach and Spleen—work together to digest and assimilate the nutrients, ideas, impressions, and experiences you take in from the outer world.

Your Stomach Official breaks down and digests the physical food as well as the experiences and ideas that you take in so that the essential nutrients can be used in service of your embodied life.

Stomach 40: Abundant Splendor

Abundant Splendor is on the outside of your leg halfway between your knee and your ankle.

Abundant Splendor gathers up the spirit of Late Summer and distributes it through your being. It stabilizes, clarifies, and nourishes your intention and supports your capacity for thoughtful, measured, and potent action.

I call on the wisdom of this point when the garden of life has gotten out of hand and too many good things are happening at the same time. It was the point that transformed one patient's wedding from a perfect storm of overwhelming details, emotions, and family members into a graceful feast of beauty, joy, and love.

When your plate is overwhelmingly full and yet there is much to be grateful for, Abundant Splendor will help you remember how to celebrate the harvest. A drop of coriander essential oil on this point will support you in receiving, digesting, and distributing the bounty of your life. It will calm you, liberate you from worry, and bring both clarity and movement.

Your Spleen Official is like a traffic director who stands at the center of a crossroads and directs the nutrients obtained from the food that the Stomach has digested. It is in charge of transforming the information you receive into potent ideas and clear thought.

Spleen 9: Yin Mound Spring

Yin Mound Spring is located in a tender spot on the inside of your leg at the bend of your knee.

In a low, damp place in a field, water accumulates, becoming stagnant and murky. The roots of the field flowers rot and invasive marsh species move in to replace them. But if a small channel opens, the water drains and is distributed into the surrounding earth. The balance of life restored, native wildflowers once again proliferate.

Yin Mound Spring is the point that opens the flow channel in you. Turn to this point when the energies in your body have become stagnant and heavy, when your mind has been invaded by worry and obsessive thoughts, or your spirit is unable to digest and assimilate the experiences of your life. Invite this point when it's time to cultivate your own growth and well-being rather than giving over your life force to others. When you find yourself invaded and strangled by the needs of others, a few drops of Centaury flower essence on this point will support you in saying no when appropriate in order to establish more healthy boundaries.

Metal

The Metal Officials—the Lung and Large Intestine—work together to help you let go of what is obsolete and devitalized in your life in order to make space to receive what is new, inspiring, and enlivening.

Your Lung Official directly regulates the rhythm of your breath and indirectly regulates the rhythm of your entire being, including heart rate, blood flow, peristalsis, and cranial rhythms. Through its regulation of the breath, this Official controls the unfolding of all your unconscious autonomic processes.

Lung 2: Cloud Gate

The Cloud Gate is at the top of your chest in a depression just below the outer edge of your clavicle.

When Autumn becomes heavy with rain and darkness wraps the edges of the day like a woven quilt, Cloud Gate opens a small passageway in the clouds so that we can catch a glimpse of the expanse beyond. After loss, depression, oppression, and death, Cloud Gate clears a way for the soul to move on, to prepare for the next stage in the journey of life.

This Metal point opens your lungs and allows you to breathe more freely. It invites you to rest in the spaciousness of grief and to rediscover your faith in emptiness. Consider Cloud Gate when you are mourning or when your soul is shrouded in depression, confusion, or despair. Consider this point when you have forgotten your own preciousness or the preciousness of others.

Your Large Intestine Official is like a good father who encourages you to leave behind your heavy suitcase of memorabilia, old books, torn clothing, and other extraneous stuff so that you can move unencumbered onward in your life. This Official disposes of all that you no longer need, on a physical, emotional, and spiritual level.

Large Intestine 11: Pool at the Crook

Pool at the Crook is at the bend of your elbow at the outer end of the line of the elbow crease.

Like any hidden pond or pool that you find when walking along a crooked path in the forest, this point is a gathering place for spirits and ghosts. We come here to help these lost beings find their resting place and help the soul let go of what it no longer needs to carry. This point allows you to release grief, trauma, and outmoded holding patterns.

Pool at the Crook opens you to your depths and allows the life force to flow. It is a point of release for both acute and chronic holding patterns. It brings Metal's medicine of deep surrender. On a physical level, this point can help relieve the discomfort of an acute sore throat and laryngitis. On an emotional level, it calms agitation and relieves tightness and oppression in the chest. On a spirit level, a drop of Rock Water flower essence on this point is like coming across an unexpected sacred spring with the power to cool, clear, and renew your life force.

Conception Vessel

Conception Vessel 15: Dove Tail

The Conception Vessel meridian runs down the front center of the torso and is the Sea of Yin Energy within you. The point Conception Vessel 15: Dove Tail is located on this line just below the lower tip of your breastbone.

Dove Tail is the mother point of the Heart Protector. It allows you to directly access, raise, and gather the wisdom of the pericardium. It clears and protects the heart in the face of emotional turmoil, uncertainty, and change.

I turn to the wisdom of this point when a patient is experiencing an emotional impasse, especially when he or she is struggling with the opposing impulses to be both vulnerable and remain safe. Dove Tail offers support when a person needs to hold the tension between trusting the self while trusting another, feeling the joy of love and the grief of loss, desiring connection while longing for protection. Dove Tail is a point of resolution and synthesis. Here, at the center of the chest, contradictions dovetail and converge.

When you are recovering from loss or betrayal, Dove Tail will bring a sense of forgiveness, acceptance, and release. When you are dealing with intimacy issues, relationship-related states of anxiety and worry, as well as feelings of overwhelm and hysteria, this point will bring a sense of trust and calm.

Governing Vessel

Governing Vessel 20: One Hundred Meetings

The Governing Vessel meridian runs down the back along your spine and is considered the Sea of Yang Energy within you. The point GV 20: One Hundred Meetings is located on this line in a small dip at the center top of your head.

One Hundred Meetings is located at the highest point of your body. It is the opening where the starlight from the Milky Way was poured into you at the time of your conception and it is through this point that your shen will fly back to the stars at the moment of your death.

On a physical level, this point helps to relieve headaches, sleepiness, heaviness in the head, as well as dizziness and brain fog. On an emotional level, it can help with feelings of depression, sadness, hyperactivity, and an inability to relax. On the level of spirit, this point helps you align your life with your authentic Tao. Touch this point when you need to get in touch with your inner compass. Invite the spirit of this point to assist you when you feel you have gone off the track of your destiny and you feel uninspired in your daily life. Visualize a gossamer thread of silk extending upward from One Hundred Meetings all the way to your personal North Star, watch your dreams, and open to the messages of Heaven.

Five Basic Alchemical Healing Protocols

When applying the essential oils and flower essences indicated for these treatments, the medicinals should be used in undiluted form. Place a drop or drops of the medicinal on a cotton swab or your fingertip and apply directly to the designated points. Hold the swab or your finger on the point for a minimum of thirty seconds to one minute to allow the point to absorb the energetic of the oil or flower essence. I've found that cotton swabs work best with flower essences due to their watery nature, and often I apply the essential oil drops directly to the points from the dropper and then apply finger pressure to the point. Avoid touching your fingers directly to the bottle or applicator to prevent contamination.

Treatment for Shock

Emotional shock leaves your body jangled and destabilized and your psychic nerve endings fried. Your shen flies out of your heart and you feel "out of it," disoriented, and confused. This treatment helps root your shen, calm your nerves, and settle your emotions after a family crisis or argument, unexpected news, a minor accident, or even when you experience excess joy and excitement after falling in love, getting engaged, or having a baby. It can help relieve shakiness and anxiety when preparing for an important presentation at work or an intimate gathering with friends. As a side effect of rooting the shen, the treatment can also relieve restlessness at night, help you fall asleep when you are overstimulated, or get back to sleep after waking from a dream.

Medicinals: Rose Essential Oil and Rock Rose Flower Essence

Spirit Points:

- 1 drop of Rose EO to Heart 7: Spirit Gate
- 3 drops of Rock Rose FE to Gall Bladder 13: Root of the Spirit
- 1 drop of Rose EO to Conception Vessel 15: Dove Tail

Imaginal Practice: As you apply the essence and the oil, visualize the Body Felt Sense feeling of shock being absorbed and transformed by the Earth and the birds of the shen settling back into the waiting nest of your heart. Once you have applied the medicinals to the points, rest quietly for at least five minutes and practice the Heart Meditation from chapter 4.

Treatment for Clarity of Mind

When your inner data processor overloads, your brain circuits clog, and your mind is filled with fuzz and fog, this treatment reboots your mental-emotional body back into smooth working order. It helps you move the sludge of trivia coming in from the news machine of the outer world and compute the information that is actually useful. It can help relieve overthinking and mental indigestion. In addition, it will help you recognize your own needs and responsibilities and clarify your intention when you are bombarded with other people's wants and demands. Last but not least, this combination of points and medicinals can help you transform worry—the unskillful use of your imagination—into a clear-headed response to present circumstance.

Medicinals: Coriander Essential Oil and Centaury Flower Essence

Spirit Points:

- 1 drop of Coriander EO to Small Intestine 19: Listening Palace

- 1 drop of Coriander EO to Spleen 9: Yin Mound Spring

- 3 drops of Centaury FE to Governing Vessel 20: One Hundred Meetings

Imaginal Practice: As you apply the oil and the essence, imagine a stream of light pouring down through the top of your head, washing through your entire body, carrying away stagnant thoughts and useless worries. As the light streams through you, it leaves behind a fresh, vibrant clarity like a sunlit morning after rain. Imagine a conduit of connection opening between your mind and your heart and ask yourself, "What do I need right now?" Pause, wait, and listen for the answer.

Treatment for Clearing and Protection

You walk away from a conversation with a colleague and dread creeps up your spine. The keen idea you came to discuss has lost its shimmer. You feel dull, dumb, and depressed. What just happened? Maybe you have been hit by another person's envy or unconscious anger. Although your colleague probably doesn't know he's envious or angry, the toxic energy still impacts you. This treatment will help clear and disperse toxic emotional energies, awaken your healthy instincts of self-protection, and create a semi-permeable shield of positive energy around you after a difficult interaction with another person, exposure to extreme emotion, or being in the presence of suffering. Touch these spirit points with the sacred balm of Frankincense and call on the protective wisdom of Holly before facing a challenging encounter with a critical boss, after a traumatic encounter with an angry friend, or when you need spiritual protection as you recover from addiction, emotional invasion, betrayal, or loss.

Medicinals: Frankincense Essential Oil and Holly Flower Essence

Spirit Points:

- 1 drop of Frankincense EO to Large Intestine 11: Pool at the Crook

- 1 drop of Frankincense EO to Triple Heater 6: Outer Frontier Gate

- 3 drops of Holly FE to Pericardium 8: Palace of Weariness

Imaginal Practice: Once you have completed the treatment, shake your hands and arms and then your whole body vigorously for three to five minutes. Imagine negative energies rushing out of your body, dispersing and transforming.

Treatment for Depletion, Over-work and Exhaustion

There is a good tiredness that comes after a day's work that is restored by a night of sleep. And then there is the bone tiredness that comes after intensive overuse of your inner resources—tending to a dying relative, completing an advanced course of study, or caring for a newborn baby after a difficult birth. This kind of fatigue can feel bottomless, as if your inner well will never be replenished. In these cases, the following combination of points and medicinals, along with time and rest, can help revitalize you. This is the treatment of choice for exhaustion after travel, emotional upheaval, or illness. It helps build depleted essences, supports appropriate self-care, and brings you back in touch with the strength of your inner mountain.

Medicinals: Balsam Fir Essential Oil and Rock Water Flower Essence

Spirit Points:

- 3 drops of Rock Water FE to Governing Vessel 20: One Hundred Meetings

The Alchemy of Inner Work

- 1 drop of Balsam Fir EO to Bladder 60: Kunlun Mountain

- 1 drop of Balsam Fir EO to Kidney 1: Bubbling Spring

Imaginal Practice: After completing this treatment, sit quietly for a few minutes and visualize roots growing downward from the point at the center of the soles of your feet, seeking, discovering, and absorbing the yin fluid life essences that course through the streams of the underworld. Imagine these essences rising upward from your feet, enlivening every cell in your body as you lean back into the imaginal mountain behind you and take in the gift of deep, restorative rest.

Treatment for Vision and Hope

As you move forward with your exploration of alchemy, you will encounter moments when it feels ridiculous to imagine that the lead of your life will transform to gold or to believe that the world around you will heal. There will be days when the suffering feels too great to bear and the weight of human fear, hatred, suspicion, and greed seems to suffocate every intrepid green sprout of hope that emerges from the darkness. In these moments, how do you return to a place of wonder? How do you find your way back to the birthright of "Wow!" that is your authentic nature?

Turn to this treatment when your imagination has gone dim and the path to the future is shrouded in impenetrable clouds. This is a treatment to remember, to offer as a gift to yourself and to your friends, and to hold in your back pocket and call on as you risk the audacity of hope.

Medicinals: Bergamot Essential Oil and Gorse Flower Essence

Spirit Points:

- 1 drop of Bergamot EO to Stomach 40: Abundant Splendor

- 1 drop of Bergamot EO to Liver 14: Gate of Hope

- 3 drops of Gorse FE to Lung 2: Cloud Gate

Imaginal Practice: As you anoint these points, bring your awareness to Stomach 40: Abundant Splendor and feel the qi move upward to Liver 14: Gate of Hope. Finally, release the energy with an inhalation and exhalation as the lungs receive the benefit of the Gorse.

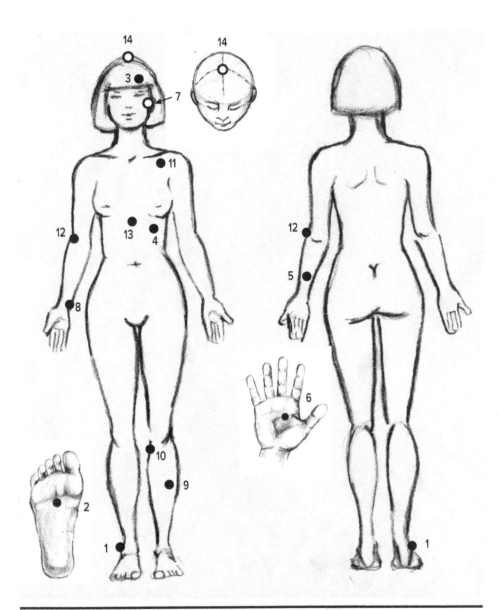

Points:

1. Bladder 60: Kunlun Mountain
2. Kidney 1: Bubbling Spring
3. Gall Bladder 13: Root of the Spirit
4. Liver 14: Gate of Hope
5. Triple Heater 6: Outer Frontier Gate
6. Pericardium 8: Palace of Weariness
7. Small Intestine 19: Listening Palace
8. Heart 7: Spirit Gate
9. Stomach 40: Abundant Splendor
10. Spleen 9: Yin Mound Spring
11. Lung 2: Cloud Gate
12. Large Intestine 11: Pool at the Crook
13. Conception Vessel 15: Dove Tail
14. Governing Vessel 20: One Hundred Meetings

Figure 10. Spirit Point Map

Chapter 11

Recovering the World of Your Dreams

Once Chuang Chou dreamt he was a butterfly, flitting and fluttering around, happy with himself and doing as he pleased. He didn't know he was Chuang Chou. Suddenly he woke up and there he was, solid and unmistakable. But he didn't know if he was Chuang Chou who had dreamt he was a butterfly, or a butterfly dreaming he was Chuang Chou.

—Chuang Tzu, Burton Watson, translator,
Chuang Tzu: Basic Writings

Living the Dream

Alchemy is the art of living in the daytime with your night eyes open. Once you enter the alchemical laboratory, the distinct delineation of the sunlit world begins to blur. Sleeping and waking are no longer opposites but rather exist on a spectrum of conscious and unconscious existence. Real and imaginal modify each other as you open to a twilight awareness quite different from the radical certainty of modern reason. To enter the laboratory, you must pass through a gate to a place you both know and have never known before. The simplest things—a cup of water, a star-shaped leaf, the scent of honeysuckle, a black crow pecking in the snow— take on meaning, become beacons, night lights, reminders of truths, and guides to next steps.

The work of modern-day alchemy is also the art of living in the night world with your daytime vision engaged. Unlike the trance states induced by a magical drumbeat, rhythmic incantation, and whirling dance of shamanic healing or the ego dissolution and spontaneously expanded states of hallucinogenic plant medicine, alchemical practices require conscious, engaged participation over time. The tools and practices of alchemy are meant to strengthen the relationship between your unbounded spiritual awareness and your unique, individuated self as well as between you and the living wisdom of the planets, plants, minerals, and beings of the world we inhabit.

In order to be effective in the alchemical laboratory and survive the disassembling challenges of transformational healing, you need to stay firmly in touch with your critical mind and capacity for rational evaluation as well as with your imagination, your body wisdom, and your heart. As an alchemist, rather than abandon the dream world to a busy morning, you steadfastly cultivate an ongoing practice of relating to your dreams. You use your conscious mind to initiate a pause. You take a few minutes to reflect. Why did my grandmother come last night covered in a blue veil, carrying a basket of starfish? Why did I dream about the old shingle house with the unhinged door banging in the wind? Why is there a kangaroo standing just outside my car window? Why do I keep coming across that same leather-bound notebook? What does it remind me of? Who gave it to me? What message do I need to write on its parchment pages?

The goal of alchemical work is not to split night and day apart or to fuse them together, but rather to resolve the paradox they present. Our work is to stay in relationship with the sun and the moon—to our thinking mind as well as our imaginal awareness—as they exist in us simultaneously. The resolution of this paradox allows you to perceive reality as it is—not a prison of matter devoid of meaning, endless bills, exhausting work, ten-second blips of disheartening media, and debilitating aches and pains, but equally not an idealistic spiritual fantasy that dead-ends in addictive numbing, fundamentalist repressive religious dogma, denial strategies, or dissociation.

In those rare moments when my day and night eyes see at the same time through the same window, time and eternity collide. When

I no longer know if I am dreaming the world or the world is dreaming me, I wake up. I remember a world I knew before I had words to describe it, a world that waits just around the corner of morning and hides behind the curtain of the night. Remembering to remember all this is the gift of dream work.

The Alchemical Attitude—Befriending the Dream

According to the Zohar, the most famous Jewish alchemical text, "A dream uninterpreted is like a letter unopened." Similarly, ancient Taoist alchemists viewed dreams as messages sent to us directly from heaven in order to help us fulfill our life mandate or destiny. C. G. Jung wrote, "Dreams are the direct expression of unconscious psychic activity." For Jung, the unconscious psyche provided the clues to understanding our psychological impasses, our obsessions, and self-sabotaging tendencies as well as our greatest life accomplishments and personal contributions. Jung believed the unconscious is the source of our life force and our connecting conduit to the transpersonal wisdom of the cosmos. From this perspective, there is no better way to honor our dreams then to tap into the source wisdom that can help us recognize our souls and foster a meaningful life.

Having worked with my own dreams and the dreams of my patients for more than thirty years, I am convinced that dreams, no matter how strange or difficult they may at first appear, almost always come in service of our healing and our wholeness. They bring us information about what we actually need to do on a daily basis to fulfill our soul's purpose. They inform our desire to do our part to further health rather than increase suffering.

The capacity to engage with dreams has been a part of human culture since the earliest times. There are anthropological accounts of indigenous people holding council meetings in the morning to discuss their dreams and assess their relevance to past and future events. It was through dreams that Jacob discovered the angels who climb between Heaven and Earth on a towering ladder, and Abraham's wife, Sarah, was protected from harm in Abimelech's harem.

From the perspective of Alchemical Healing, dream work is not a specialized practice reserved for a privileged few but rather the spiritual birthright of every person. It is an intrinsic part of a fulfilling life, one of the most reliable ways to communicate with the Self and to track the progress of your path through life.

Despite common belief, the first step in the process of relating to your dreams is not to correctly analyze the meaning of the dream, to tear it apart in order to extract its message, or to consult an authoritative text that can interpret the language of its symbols. Dream work begins by beginning to care about your dream. It begins when you take the time to reflect on its needs and desires, to feel into its atmosphere, to inhale its scent, and trace the edges of its skin. It begins when you wonder about its native terrain and the beings who inhabit its homeland. Jungian analyst James Hillman refers to this as "befriending" the dream:

> Friendship wants to keep the connection open and flowing. . . .
> Befriending the dream begins with a plain attempt to listen to
> the dream, to set down on paper or in a dream diary in its own
> words just what it says. . . . Befriending is the feeling approach
> to the dream, and so one takes care receiving the dream's feel-
> ings, as with a living person with whom we begin a relationship.

The crucial question is not "What does this dream mean?" but "What does this dream want and need?" Caring deeply about that question is the first step in making friends with your dream.

Dream Work Basics

When I work with my own dreams or the dreams of my students and patients, I always begin with the recognition that the dream may not share my conscious values or ideals, but it is unquestionably committed to my entelechy, the movement of my life toward the fulfillment of my end and the attainment of more wholeness. Even when the dream is disturbing, I always look for the edge that leads to something new, a piece I didn't know before that opens me to a larger view of myself and my life's possibilities.

In the midst of writing this book, I dreamt that Benjamin put his fist through one of my brother's paintings and punched a hole in the middle of the canvas. I woke up upset and concerned that my husband was trying to destroy my creativity. This dream came at a moment in our collaborative editorial process when Benjamin was leaning on me to step into my innate Martian Aries nature and take more risks in my writing. Over time, as I sat with the dream, I came to realize that the Benjamin of my dream, who was also a part of me, was telling me I needed to break through a self-imposed barrier to a new part of my creative process. By punching a hole in the canvas, Benjamin was trying to liberate me from the patriarchal attitudes of my artist father and brother as well as the academic constraints of the mainstream Chinese medical community, both of which I've internalized during my lifetime. As I continued to befriend this dream, I felt its life-affirming energy rush through my body, calling me to stretch beyond my own self-imposed limitations and to free up my aggression in service to my authentic voice and vision for my writing, my art, and my work as a healer.

The second thing I always try to remember when working with dreams is that only the dreamer can ultimately interpret the dream. Even the most brilliant analysis by the most seasoned expert pales in comparison to the felt sense of a shift in the dreamer's emotional body when she gets the gist of the dream. Whereas other people can offer useful insights or ask supportive leading questions, the "click" or "aha!" response in the dreamer is the most reliable indication that we've gotten the dream's most essential meaning.

When a patient dreamt she had inherited a dream home in Athens from a long-deceased great aunt and then realized that water was pouring through all the windows to form a deep turquoise pool across the entire ground floor, I was sure the dream was telling her that she needed to create a stronger boundary between herself and her extended family. There was no question in my mind that the "inheritance" she was due to receive from her wealthy parents would not be worth the invasive flooding of their emotional demands. I felt certain I had the right interpretation. Thankfully, I managed to stay quiet and curious while she worked with the dream images.

After a few minutes of silence, she spoke. "I love to swim," she said, "and as I look at that house filling with water, I realize how amazing it is that my aunt has left this place to me, not only the home but a pool that I can dive down into, a place to meet my past and the gods and goddesses hiding there." As she worked with the dream, she realized how critical it would be for her to stay in touch with the pleasure of her own body, her love of swimming, and memories of her ancestry if she were to transform the challenging aspects of her family inheritance into something that could truly support her. This experience affirmed what I already knew, and it comes back to me whenever I am tempted to rush in too quickly with a clever interpretation of another person's dream.

Another thing to remember is that a dream symbol is like a crystal with many facets. Just as a crystal offers multiple vantage points, a dream symbol allows us many approaches to an interpretation. Every viewpoint of a crystal reveals a different shape and yet each is related to the whole. Similarly, in dream work, there is no one right perspective, no one right answer. The association or interpretation that is "right" is the one that moves you, that quickens your breathing or elicits an emotion. In order to broaden the range of your associations and interpretations of dream symbols, familiarize yourself with myths, legends, and fairy tales and the universal archetypes that show up in stories told from around the world. Getting to know these ancient tales will help you recognize the beings that wander in and through your night world, making it easier for you to understand their language.

Keep your dream work manageable. Don't bite off more than you can chew. You can always come back to a powerful dream again later. I have dreams I worked with over decades and one I had as a child about a witch in a bakery that is still an active piece of my inner work. When you don't have time to work with an entire dream, don't feel pressured to rush through it. Instead, pick the part of the dream that calls to you and trust that, like a hologram, that single fragment or scene has value. It will tell you what you need to know now. "My ex-husband was taking care of three orphaned babies" or "I noticed that my silver wedding band was missing" or "I reach down into a stream of water and pull up a writhing, iridescent fish." These pieces of dreams are all letters waiting to be opened, messages ready to be delivered. Any piece of a dream is linked by a fine silken thread to the archetypal information it contains and will open you to the wisdom of the dream's wholeness.

Care about the beings in your dreams. Relate to them as you would a friend. Pause as you would before a place of natural beauty. An apple tree. A small brown mouse. A bald eagle flying overhead. Your old high school principal. Having lunch with the president. An aging ballerina leaping over a fire. Ask questions. Converse with the people and creatures who show up. Take time to listen to their replies. Why have you come? What do you want me to know? What gift are you bringing? What gift are you asking me for?

When you listen to another person's dream, you do not need to fix anything, give advice, or help the dreamer unravel the dream. You are a witness creating a safe space for the work, supporting the process with your presence. Again, ask questions. Be with another person's dream as if it were your own but always remember that you are not that person. Your gift is simply caring enough to let the dream be told.

Last but not least, remember that like any authentic spiritual teacher, the unconscious has a sense of humor and loves to play tricks. Take time to catch the puns, appreciate the poetry, revel in the riddles and divine humor of the dream weaver. When you dream you are eating a bowl of green peas, consider whether you need to make someone a peace offering. And if you arrive at a friend's party wearing a black and white jumpsuit, you may need to take a leap into the shades of grey in your relationship. When you wake up thinking, "That was the craziest dream I ever had, just a bunch of nonsense," you can be sure there is a bit of hidden gold that should not be thrown away.

Getting Started

Dreams benefit us even if we don't do anything with them. Simply having a dream benefits your body and your mind. Even when you don't remember a dream, the dream is restoring balance to your nervous system and helping your psyche integrate the events of the previous day. However, the practice of actively remembering your dreams greatly amplifies their benefit as it allows you to bring their messages to conscious awareness. Writing the dream down in a dream journal, recording a symbol or image in a drawing, or sharing the dream with another person imprints its message into a material form that allows you to effectively work with it.

The next step is connecting the dream to events in your current life. This act takes your dream work to another level and it is where the alchemy actually begins. There are three ways you can make this connection: The first is through feeling into the general atmosphere of the dream. The second is by making associations to its images. The third is through an alchemical practice called Active Imagination.

Feeling into the atmosphere of a dream is like sitting next to a friend without talking. You don't need words to know if your friend is happy, excited, or having a rough time. Because you care, you notice the cues—the way your friend is breathing, the expression on her face, how her fingers twist the hem of a sleeve.

To know how your dream is feeling, take time to pay attention. What happens in your body when you go back into the dream? What emotions come? Does your chest release or tighten? Do you feel drawn closer or pushed away? Does your breathing quicken or slow down? All this information will give you clues to how the dream is feeling and what it wants you to know about something happening in your life right now.

The next dream practice, working with associations, is like writing a poem or solving a jigsaw puzzle. Let all the thoughts and images that rise up in relationship to the dream float freely through your mind. Jot them down on paper and keep gathering associations until a picture begins to form.

In working with associations, you go back into the dream and once again notice how you feel. But this time ask into the feelings themselves. What does this emotion or body sensation remind me of? When did I last feel that way and with whom did I feel that way? Or take one of the significant images from the dream and consider what it relates to. There is no need to be rational or to force it to make sense. For example, the kangaroo outside my car window belongs in Australia, not Maine. I'm surprised that she has come here, this large furry beast carrying her baby in her pouch. The associative words that come are: mother, on the move, marsupial, magic. She surprises me. She makes me laugh. But she also makes me nervous. And then, click! I get what the dream is up to. I am thrilled that my daughter is going to have a baby. Something that once seemed so distant is now right here. Suddenly, I am going to be a grandmother! I'm happy and nervous at the same time. Along with my excitement, I am concerned about the responsibility, about being weighed down. Am I ready to take this on? Can I be there for my daughter and grandchild in the midst of my already full and busy life? The kangaroo has come to give me some new information, to show me something about being nurturing while maintaining my wildness.

Active Imagination is the most advanced of the three methods of alchemical dream work. In this practice, you use the tools of alchemy—imaginal sight, Inner Sensing, deep listening—to bring the images of your dream to life by relating to them. You can do this practice in an hour or over a period of days, months, or years, but to do it effectively you need to shut out the noise of the outer world and enter the meditation space of your inner laboratory. Once there, you need some way to record your conversation with your dream being, whether in writing, drawing, movement, or song.

Active Imagination is like transcribing an interview where both the questions and the answers matter. I ask the kangaroo, "Why are you standing there outside my car window?" And I hear her say, "Because I know something you need to know too." I reply, "Okay, so what's that?" And then I hear, "I know how to be on the move and take care of a baby at the same time." She winks at me and sticks her furry face through the open window. I smell her musky smell. I feel intimidated by her big, yellow teeth and shiny, sniffing nose. "I'm not sure I'm ready to take you on," I say. "It's too late," she replies. "It's happening. I'm here and I'm getting in your car!" Uh oh. I get it. She wants to be part of me. I ask her, "So how do I do this thing with the new baby?" And she says, "Easy! Keep your sense of humor. Don't look back. Stay easy on your feet with one hand in your pocket and you'll be fine. I can do it and so can you!" I get a feeling in my body that makes me laugh. I say, "I guess a dose of kangaroo medicine is just what I need!"

The last benefit of dreaming comes when you understand what the dream wants or needs from you and you respond by taking an action step or making a real change in your life. You can use Active Imagination to get at the particulars or you can watch where your feelings or associations lead you. What change of behavior, perception, or attitude is needed now? What new way of being? What new possibility is ready to emerge? Once the necessary change becomes clear to you, resolve to take an actual step in the direction of the dream's request by way of a small symbolic ritual or a major shift in behavior.

For me, it was the kangaroo's big yellow teeth in my Active Imagination process that stood out. Fierce, hungry, and scary, ready to bite even when she was smiling. Her teeth are not nice or pretty, but they get the job done. Those teeth are telling me to keep a grip on my life, not to get mired down in trying to be all-caring and motherly. I'm too old for that. My fur is too thick and dusty from travel. But I do have a job to support this courageous little human as she arrives at this uncertain, tumultuous time on the planet. As a grandmother, I will need to maintain my freedom, fierceness, and humor while helping her find her way and purpose. As a ritual, I'm going to find myself a furry sling to carry this new baby in. At the first opportunity, I'm taking her on a walkabout under the stars. Although so many of the animals of our day world are dying, the night world is still filled with wondrous, mysterious creatures that desperately need our care. Working with dreams will be part of the legacy I leave her.

What If You Don't Dream?

Many of my patients and students tell me they can't do dream work because they don't dream. But the truth is that everyone dreams. Even dogs and cats dream, and so do whales, dolphins, elephants, and foxes. We don't know about snakes, stones, or trees, but if you ask me, I'd say yes, definitely, they dream in their own way.

Many people do not remember their dreams or remember so few that they forget about them completely. If this is the case for you, I encourage you to try the following suggestions. Most people I work with find that they start remembering their dreams quite readily once they implement these simple strategies.

Keep a dream journal and a pen right next to your bed. Or if you prefer using your phone or laptop, have it within reach. You can type your dreams right onto your device or record them vocally. Any way you can get your dreams down is fine. Just having something there, ready to write or record on, is a message to the dream weaver that you are really serious about staying in communication.

Set the intention to remember your dreams before you go to sleep. Sometimes, it can help to write a question on paper and put it under your pillow. In the morning, take a few minutes to wake up slowly. As soon as you move your physical body, the memory of your dream begins to dissipate, so stay as still as you can and ask, "What happened last night?" Then get something down in your journal. Don't be concerned if you only remember a word or a feeling or a single image. These bits are like fine silver hooks that can eventually link you to the larger net of your dream weavings.

Spirit Bear and the Ad Man's Alchemical Healing Journey

The case I describe here is a composite of treatments that took place over the course of a decade. It shows how the alchemical tools I discuss in this and previous chapters work in actual practice, including elemental associations, imaginal sight, archetypes, Inner Sensing, flower essences, and dream work. It presents difficult, controversial, and potentially triggering issues that show up regularly in my practice and in our current culture, including infertility, infidelity, depression, addiction, and the destructive effects of the objectification of women on the feminine and masculine aspects of the soul.

There are practitioners who might have drawn back from working with this particular patient and I recognize there may be readers who find his story personally and politically objectionable. In fact, in the years we worked together, there were times when I was deeply troubled by the way my patient treated the women in his life.

I spoke openly to my patient about my feelings of discomfort and upset in response to his behavior and attitudes. I believe that our ongoing, radically honest, and mutually respectful dialogue were key components of the alchemy that took place between us and ultimately, to a significant piece of healing for him. In the end, I felt that our work together presented an opportunity that transcended both our personal identities. Together, we touched some of the deepest, most raw wounds of our time, including the denigration of the divine Feminine, the divorce between the principles of yin and yang, and the toxic masculinity that dominates our modern culture. Despite certain hesitations, I present this case as a reminder that in order to discover gold, we must begin with lead. Who we may become begins with who we are. The long, convoluted, and always surprising path between now and then is the journey of Alchemical Healing.

When this man arrived in my practice, he was already a senior executive at a top New York City advertising agency. Tall, gangly, hardworking, financially ruthless, and practical, he also had a quicksilver wit and wide-ranging curiosity about everything from fly fishing to French wine, basketball to Zen meditation. Yet underneath his charming warmth, self-assurance, and agile mind, I felt a hesitancy, a holding back at the edge of his easy masculinity.

During our initial interview, he revealed to me, as if in passing, that his mother had taken a poorly tested medication while she was pregnant with him. He was born with a kink in his genetic sequencing that resulted in complete sterility. By the time he entered puberty, he already understood that he would never be able to father a child of his own blood.

Along with this congenital reproductive issue, his long spine, low back pain, groaning voice, powerful ambition, and deeply hidden anxiety about his own potency reflected my patient's resonance with the Water Element. Related to the Season of Winter and the

Emotion Fear, Water is also related to the quality and storage of our inner and outer resources. These resources include our ancestral life essences, which endow us with the capacity to pass on our genetic inheritance to future generations. Water regulates our most primal drives of reproduction and survival. It compels us to seek and bank away sufficient reserves to keep us going through lean, cold times and to gather strength and resilience from rest and gestation. I quickly recognized that my patient's deepest wounds resided at this level. As it turned out, he was very concerned about having enough—enough money in the bank, enough status in his firm, enough security for his retirement and, as was revealed over time, enough women to prove he was really a potent and legitimate man.

At first, I focused on his physical symptoms—the back pain, the knee pain, the restless leg that woke him in the night—symptoms that were all also related to Water in traditional Chinese medicine. But as I worked with Water Element acupuncture points to relieve his physical symptoms, the soul-level issues began to emerge from deeper levels. I became aware of a persistent Body Felt Sense that there was more hidden, a feeling of pressure when he spoke, of some-thing waiting under the surface. There was the hesitancy, as if he was about to say something but then stopped. I was struck by the way he played with his keyring or looked out the window when I questioned him about his relationships. I was aware that pieces of the story weren't adding up.

I decided to introduce him to flower essences as a way to augment our work with needles. He was skeptical but said that because he found my various practices entertaining, he'd give the "fairy flowers" a try. The first flower essence I suggested was Rock Rose, my essence of choice for Water and one I often turn to for healing trauma and dredging up what has been buried beneath the surface. Although he had not made a big deal about it, I felt that he was carrying signifi-cant trauma from his mother's use of drugs during his gestation and his subsequent sterility. Then there was the feeling he was hiding things—secrets, emotions—below the surface of his self-assured per-sona. I thought of the seeds of the rock rose plant buried beneath the soil, surviving wildfires and floods, waiting to sprout again when the conditions were favorable. The flower fit, so I made it a part of the treatment. A few weeks later, the deeply buried seeds began to sprout.

The stories of the sexual encounters, love affairs, and romantic exploits came slowly. At first, drop by drop. Then, in increasing detail. In his cautious, calculating way, he was testing me. How deeply could his Water Element trust me? Would I judge or reject him?

As the state of his physical spine improved, the spine of his subtle body also strengthened. Gradually, it seemed he could stand up straighter in our conversations. He could show more of himself. He could take the risk of coming out of hiding and telling someone the whole truth of his situation. The stories came over months and years, threaded in with reports on business deals, Winter vacations, frequent urination, sciatica. Gradually, his desperate sexual exploits and their exhausting effects on his body and soul became the focus of our work.

There were stories of meetings, trysts, flirtations, and innuendo-laden conversations. The thrill of the hunt, the magical moment when he lured in his prey, the shameful inability to perform, and then the curt terminations of connection. He told me of women he picked up during happy hour cocktails, quick kisses under tiki bar palm trees, heart-to-hearts around pools, fire pits, or on flights to Los Angeles. I heard of further exploits while grabbing a sandwich on 57th Street, on the beach, the ski mountain, the safari. All the incredible happy endings after well-earned massages. Long distance cyber encounters. "Serious" relationships with executives from other firms, in other cities, other states, other countries. Arizona. Alaska. Boston. Miami. Canada. Switzerland. Brazil. The U. K.

Yet, there was never a final trophy. No woman was really "right," the one to stay with, to commit to, to dive down deep with and truly know.

In the end, after the encounters, the affairs, the two marriages and divorces, he returned home to his solo life, his luxurious but empty midtown apartment, and his growing sense that he was missing out on some critically important aspect of life. It took time and patience on my part, but after many conversations, many dreams, many repeated explanations, my patient finally became curious about what (besides momentary sexual pleasure and brief ego gratification) might drive his compulsion. Eventually, he admitted, he was tiring of it. Despite his genuine enjoyment of women's company, the thrill of the sexual conquest was gone. The hunt was losing its "zing." The adrenaline no longer rushed. The Viagra no longer did the trick. The whole thing had become predictable and tiring. The truth was that, like all addictions, his sex addiction was robbing him of exactly what it promised: the renewal, creativity, and healing of shared pleasure and the enlivening warmth and support of relatedness.

The realization that what we have been desperately searching for in the outer world may actually be a quest for something we have lost in our own being comes as a shock. Everything conscious in us at first rejects this idea. The "out there" is so infinitely seductive that it takes an act of enormous faith, will, or grace to tear our gaze away from the endless array of people and stuff, to bring focus to bear on the interior, to the realm of our own soul. And yet, from an alchemical perspective, inner work truly begins with this turning around of the light, this reversal of awareness, with asking the central question, "Who am I?" Once we recognize that the shimmering glamour and fascination of external phenomena are reflections of something necessary, something compelling, something divine that dwells within rather than without, nothing is ever quite the same.

For my patient, the moment of reversal came during a fishing trip in the wilderness of northern British Columbia. Although we had been discussing archetypes for some time in our sessions and he intellectually understood the concept, it wasn't until a chance meeting at the edge of a rushing river that he got an embodied understanding that the archetypes are real, that they live outside but also inside of him.

I could tell something had shifted as soon as I saw him in the waiting room after he got back from his trip. He seemed more present, sobered and yet, at the same time, vibrating with excitement.

"Do I have a story for you!" he exclaimed when we sat down face to face in the treatment room. "What a trip!"

I settled back in my chair, took a deep breath, sunk down into my body, and prepared to listen. Here is what he said:

"Picture this . . . nothing but forest, mountains, sky. Late September. Days growing shorter but still warm. Afternoon sunlight pouring down like honey. I'm standing in the river. Salmon everywhere. Some fighting their way upstream to spawn, some already done, losing strength, dying, floating belly up in the water or washed up on the bank. I'm standing there under this big blue arching sky. Looking up, I see the bald eagles circling, getting ready to dive for the fish. Life, death, sex, rebirth, it's all there, the smell of fresh spawn mixed with the stink of decaying fish flesh. The whole circle of life right in front of me, full circle. I can't believe I'm really there in the middle of it.

"That's when it happened. I hear something rustling in the brush behind me. I turn around. Twelve feet away from me. Maybe less. Standing straight up on her back legs. Three hundred pounds at least. Probably more. All white. No joke. An all-white she-bear! Looking right at me. I mean, eye to eye. She sees me. I see her. That's when I get it. It's her. It's the archetype, the Goddess herself. Coming out of the forest, coming down to the river. Coming to meet me.

"Right then. Everything stops. She can take me down with one blow. My life is in her hands. I feel something give way. I'm tunneling down her eyes. She's looking at me, in me, through me. I can die at any moment but I'm not afraid. I feel something like a creaking door in my chest. I'm all hers. I'm wide open. The ache is unbelievable, but I don't want it to stop.

"I get it. I'm completely okay. She won't do anything to hurt me. There's nothing I need. Nothing I don't have. Everything inside of me lets go. I'm safe. I'm cared for. I have enough. I feel a peace I've never felt before. And all I can feel is love.

"We stand there like that. Just looking at each other. I don't know how much time. Maybe thirty seconds. Maybe a hundred years. And then it's done. Over. I get the message. She knows it and so do I. I'm back in time. An eagle swoops down and grabs a fish. The world is breathing again. My legs feel like cooked noodles. She turns away. She's gone. Back into the forest. The guide boat drifts towards me. It's time to go."

I looked at him and he looked back. No twiddling fingers. No averted gaze. For the first time, I felt he was seeing me as a whole person, seeing my feminine wisdom with affection, appreciation, and respect. Until his encounter with the bear, it had all been a game for him. It was as if he were humoring me rather than taking our work seriously. He hadn't really taken in that his compulsion to seduce, trap, and dominate women came from a feeling of his own power-lessness in the face of the Feminine, in the face of life and death. He hadn't yet taken in the destructive effects his behavior was having on his own well-being and the women he came in contact with. And it hadn't yet really sunken in that it was only through an embodied encounter with this other—this divine Feminine who was also a part of his own Self—that he could heal from the rage he felt toward his mother for her unwitting betrayal of his masculinity and his shame around the inability to father a child from his own seed.

"You got it," I said. "That bear. She could have taken you down with one swipe of her paw and yet she showed you only love. All you needed to do was to really see her."

When I needled the spirit point on the bottom of his feet that day, it was a way of celebrating and tattooing into his body the feel-ing of rootedness and stability that came from his encounter with the bear. Through this alchemical meeting, he had opened to the Bubbling Spring of his own spiritual resources and his own imaginal sight. After years of repeated suggestions on my part, he finally got it. The "she" he had been relentlessly pursuing in the outer world was the "she" inside of him—the fullness of his authentic emotions, his capacity for actual embodied eroticism, and his deep caring for the beauty of life.

Our work changed after that. There was a different quality to our conversations. I felt less seductiveness in the field between us, more warmth and easy affection. I felt I could let my guard down when we hugged at the end of a session. My patient became more interested in the needs of his own body. He started doing yoga, drinking less, eating differently. He was able to relax more deeply on the treatment table. He began talking about retiring from his job, not pushing so hard, doing things differently.

"I went out with a buddy last night. Had a couple of drinks. There were some women at the next table. One tall, nice, wearing tight jeans, with that kind of dark red hair I like. I knew I could have her. I knew just what to do to reel her in. But when I felt into my body the way you've showed me how to do, I felt the way it feels after a good rainstorm, calm and peaceful. None of that pressure inside, no need to chase her, catch her like a fish in a net. I didn't need to do anything. I could just sit back, enjoy the vibe, the conversation, the place. So that's what I did. It felt great. A real relief.

"When she got up to leave, she looked my way. I knew she would. She smiled at me and I smiled back. And it was right there. It was understood. That energy between us. We both knew. It felt good. And her smile. And knowing, knowing and feeling. It was enough.

"I'm beginning to get it. This isn't about some woman who is going to make it better, who is going to fix the part of me that was broken. It isn't about the chase, the hunt, the adrenaline rush that blots out the sadness and the pain. It's just about me being there, wherever I am, knowing I'm okay. Leaning back into my life and knowing I can let certain things take their own course.

"I guess I've been angry at her all this time, angry that she didn't listen to her body, that she took those drugs, that she didn't have the sense, the animal in her didn't question . . . well, whatever. It's done. And I can move on."

A few months later, he came in excited. "You won't believe this dream," he began. "No. Really. Sometimes, I am just blown away by this stuff. I was in a bordello in some town in Wyoming. You know the kind they have in old Western movies. Ornate furniture. Red velvet curtains. Whiskey. Cigars. Honkytonk music. Lots of pretty girls in see-through lingerie gliding in and out of open doorways. But instead of feeling good, turned on, excited, I feel something tight in the pit of my stomach. I know I'm not there for the pretty girls. I'm there for the Madame.

"I walk down a long hallway and then enter a room lit with lots of candles. There is a screen and behind it, I see a couch. Lots of pillows. Long legs. Big breasts. Lips. Silk and satin. Gorgeous. Lush. Big. She's it. The real deal. And not to be toyed with.

"She beckons me to come closer. I approach. And then I pause.

"This one . . . you don't mess with her. This woman I thought at first was a prostitute is the Goddess herself. She's the one you've been trying to talk to me about. And the real joke . . . I get it now . . . it was her all along. All those girls. All those women. Each one has a little bit of her in them. That's what I was chasing. But, me, I was prostituting my own soul. I wasn't paying attention to the 'she' inside me. She's the one I have to listen to. She's the one who has to come first. And here's the real news: I no longer have a choice. I'm her guy. She's the one I have to answer to. As far as other women, well, we'll see what happens with all that down the line."

Not long after this dream, my patient began to talk about radically changing his life, retiring after forty years from his high-pressure job, selling his apartment and living somewhere closer to nature. He started taking his meditation practice more seriously and began reading some recent writing on the effects of early trauma on brain physiology and addiction. After many years, our work together began to wind down. We said our formal goodbye a few days before he celebrated his retirement and began packing up to move to a small place, somewhere north, on a river.

Like many of my patients who move on after long years of exploration, I have not heard from him since our last meeting. I do not know whether his inner alchemy continues or whether he has forgotten about his commitment to his marriage with the woman within. I do not know whether he lives alone, has found a partner or has picked up again on his compulsive sexual exploits and addiction.

When I think about him, I feel a sadness and also a deep gratitude. Through our work together, I was forced to accept my own powerlessness. I could not force him with my judgment, my will, or my needles to change his behavior. Instead, through a kind of fierce honesty and hard-won empathy, we gradually got to know each other as flawed and vulnerable human beings. I had to face the discomfort of my own shadowy feelings of contempt and superiority and continuously ask whether I was in integrity with my own values in continuing to work with him. He had to find the courage to come out of hiding and bear his soul to another. In the process, alchemy happened. Through the sacredness of the relationship that constellated between us, the seed of a new possibility was planted in the dark soil of the world soul.

Part Three

Discovering Gold

Chapter 12

The Alchemy of Gender

Individuality is direction within continual change. What makes us
individuals is not the immutability of our properties but the conscious
awareness of the continuity of meaningful and consistent transformation.

—Lama Anagarika Govinda, *The Inner Structure*
of the I Ching

The Inner Partner

I began working with Amy while she was in training to become a psychotherapist. She was an intrepid explorer, hungry to understand her own terrors and passions, to plunge the depths of her own psyche. She eventually completed her studies and met a lovely man who became her devoted, successful husband. Somewhere along the way, as a happily married woman with a young child, Amy disappeared for a while into her life.

When she returned, it was to tell me that she wakes in the night with her heart pounding. In Amy's dreams, her college boyfriend, a drug dealer and an addict, a lawless street fighter who abandoned her repeatedly, is stalking her. Several times a week, he returns, smelling of smoke and leather and the open road, to whisk her away on his black Harley.

She wakes up restless, confused, frustrated, and unsatisfied, wondering if she needs to leave her marriage. "I feel terrible," she says. "I love my husband. Why do I keep dreaming of Bobby?"

Gradually, over months of conversation and courageous self-reflection, Amy comes to understand that this dream is a symbolic story of her soul's deepest longing. Rather than a calling to leave her husband and young child and ride off onto the open road, the dream is an invitation to something much more daunting: a challenge to return to her own inner work, to fall in love with the wild, fearless adventuring part of her Self that she abandoned when she became a wife and mother. To grow closer to her own wholeness, her task is to take back the disowned parts of her Self that she projected on to Bobby. Despite its disturbing nature, Amy's dream, like all dreams, has come in service of her healing.

The Bobby who comes to Amy in her dreams is not exactly the same Bobby she dated in college, and yet he carries some of the same dangerous, irresistible allure. In particular, he has some very specific yang, stereotypically masculine traits—reckless adventurousness, power, freedom, and bad-boy wildness—that Amy disowned in her conscious personality. Bobby is an emissary of Amy's Self. He is the messenger, the guide, who has come to lead her through the wilderness in the search for her lost pieces. From an alchemical perspective, Bobby is Amy's mystical sibling, her inner soul partner, the one who holds the key to her inner laboratory.

This inner partner may appear in an embodied outer relationship, projected onto a person you become entranced or obsessed with, even fall in love with and marry, or it may show up as a fantasy involvement—a movie character or famous personality you fixate on or, as in the case with Amy, a seductive or disturbing dream figure. In fact, the soul partner does exist, not entirely in the outer or inner world, but in the mutable inner/outer realm of the subtle body. It lives in the space between self and other, matter and spirit, he and she. It is here where you must go to truly discover who this partner is.

Myths, legends, and ancient texts describe the archetype of the soul partner in different ways: a magical child, a spouse, a sibling, king, queen, a crippled warrior, fool, or long-lost friend. This mystical other shows up as the Egyptian goddess Isis, who gathers up the dismembered parts of her lover Osiris in order to repair his body and bring him back to life; as Catherine's brooding brother Heathcliff, who alternately inspires and torments her in Emily Brontë's gothic tale *Wuthering Heights*; as Rhett Butler, who ultimately forces Scarlett O'Hara to find her own determination and resiliency; as Penelope, the wife who waits and weaves until her sea-faring husband Odysseus makes his way home to heal and receive her love. No matter the form, the inner partner always comes as a guide to greater wholeness. It acts as a bridge between our limited conscious ego identity and the vast spaciousness of the Self. From an alchemical perspective, this movement toward our own wholeness is the ultimate purpose not only of any relationship but of our entire life. It is the basis of the greatest of all the alchemical mysteries—the coniunctio or inner marriage.

The Alchemical Marriage

The union, dissolution, and reunion of opposites to form a new, more elegant, and enduring wholeness is the organizing principal of all alchemical work. Whether you are an acupuncturist working with the ebb and flow of yin and yang in the body, an artist working with the interplay of light and dark in a painting, an herbalist creating a balanced medicinal tincture, or a lover bearing the rhythmic pulsation of connection and disconnection in a human relationship, you are in the domain of the alchemical marriage.

An alchemical relationship that supports this kind of reorganization—the rejoining of separated parts and the reuniting of opposites to form a new wholeness—is possible when your psychic energies are activated as were Amy's by her dreams of Bobby. This activation can be felt as a quality of excitation, a passion, a persistent curiosity, an inspiration, or an intensification of focus. You can recognize it by a feeling of desire, hatred, strangeness, or love, a disturbance of your inner equilibrium, a thickening of the emotional atmosphere. It may come as the nagging tug of a project left undone as it did for one patient of mine whose depression finally lifted when he returned to painting after twenty years away from his studio. It may come as a forbidden attraction that shakes the foundation of your marriage as it did for a friend who was completely undone by her passionate longing for her son's football coach until she realized that he represented a long-denied need to cultivate her own physical strength and unleash her competitive drive. Or it may show up as a seemingly senseless obsession with a politician, a character in a television series, or a charismatic pop star as it did for one of my students who couldn't stop watching Beyoncé's "Listen" music video until he realized he needed to find his own voice and take his own talents seriously.

At these disrupting moments of fascination, passion, despair, longing, and heightened emotion, it is crucial not to be tricked into looking for resolution outside yourself, by impulsively abandoning a relationship, joining a cult, leaving a job, or moving to a new country, but rather to look within. At these critical junctures, according to the wisdom of ancient alchemy, your *sorora mystica*, your mystical soul partner, is knocking at the door of your inner laboratory, calling you to reverse the handle of the stars and come back to your inner work. Before rushing into externalized action, alchemy invites you to pause, to look within, to listen to the messages of your body and your dreams, to wait to see where the journey of Tao is actually leading and then to dare to follow the bold calling of the Self.

Anima/Animus

In the early 1900s, C. G. Jung brought the idea of the alchemical soul partner and the inner marriage into modern psychological discourse through his development of the concept of the *syzygy*, the pairing of the archetypal gender opposites: yin/yang and he/she. Through his ongoing exploration of myth, art and religious ritual, his own psyche, and his clinical work with patients, Jung came to believe that the syzygy exists in every person in the form of an inner partner that is the psychic complement to their outer conscious gender identity. The inner partner, while less accessible to conscious awareness than our ego, plays an essential role in the development of our psychology. It has a significant influence on the way we feel inside, the life choices we make, and the behavior patterns that fix our personalities and draw us toward our destinies.

In keeping with his time, Jung believed that the traits associated with gender were universal, innate, and archetypal based on biology. In his view, a healthy person born with male anatomy, XY chromosomes, and a penis would grow to view himself as a man and have a conscious orientation to behaviors and attitudes identified by his family and culture as masculine. Similarly, a healthy person born with female anatomy, XX chromosomes, and a vagina would grow to view herself as a woman and consciously orient to traits identified by her family and culture as feminine. As he developed his theory, Jung assumed that the complementary inner soul partner would automatically carry the attitudes and energies of the gender opposite to our innate biological reproductive anatomy, chromosomal make-up, and dominant sex hormones.

According to Jung, every biological man has an innate yang phallic drive related to the nature and function of his sexual anatomy that forms a foreground aspect of his ego identity. However, he also has an inner opposite, a recessive yin soul partner or complementary "inner woman," which Jung called the *anima*, who carries qualities associated with female anatomy, such as receptivity and inwardness. The anima is an archetype that Jung believed is an inborn aspect of the male psyche, so she expresses certain collectively recognized feminine qualities and general cultural assumptions about women. The anima is also personal and reflects a man's individual impressions and unique experiences with women he has early, formative contact with—mothers, caregivers, sisters, and family friends. At her best, the anima gives a man the capacity for self-reflection, receptivity, patience, gestation, and process. She helps him to care about his feelings, his body needs, and the eros function—his capacity for relationship and intimate connection. At her worst, when ignored or unrelated to, she draws him away from authentic connection with self and other, into moody withdrawal, regressive longings, paralysis and silence, instability, hypersensitivity, self-pity, and cloying sentimentality.

To complete his theory, Jung went on to say that every biological woman is born with an innate yin receptivity, gestational capacity, and depth of feeling related to the nature and function of her genitality. In addition, she also has an inner opposite, a recessive yang soul partner or "inner man" he called the *animus*, who carries the attributes and drives associated with the male sexual anatomy. A healthy animus gives a woman the capacity for phallic drive, initiative, goal orientation, penetrating thought, and effective outward action. He helps her articulate her ideas and values and regulate her *logos* function—her integrity of mind and word. At his worst, the animus incites a rigid, judgmental attitude in a woman that leads her to argue about things she knows very little about. A negative animus-driven woman can become picky, critical, bossy, and intrusive and ends up alienating the people she most desires to be close with.

The anima and animus can act as background supports to the ego and invaluable guides to the Self, or they can become possessive tricksters who lure us away from our own best nature and sabotage our outer relationships. According to Jung, the determining factor is our consciousness, our ability to become aware of the inner partner's presence, to recognize when it is activated, to relate to it with respect, and to care about its needs and desires. Our conscious awareness transforms the inner partner from a potentially dangerous demon into something almost divine, a kind of angel who travels by our side.

Until we learn to consciously relate to the inner partner, it will continue to tug at our emotions and instincts and undermine our plans by pulling us into relationships and actions that are at odds with our conscious values, commitments, and beliefs. For example, if Amy had not been able to recognize that Bobby was an expression of her own adventurous, rebellious nature and not an actual desire for connection to a dangerous man, she might have taken a self-destructive outer action. Instead, she came to understand that the Bobby in her dream needed her to relate to him and to truly care about his needs and values, which were different from her husband's and her own. Over time, she developed a relationship to this inner other. Supported and guided by him, she began traveling to conferences and workshops on her own. She made time to develop her writing and share it on her website. She put energy into growing a unique and successful private practice. In this way, she came back to her own authentic nature as an edgy, risk-taking healer while maintaining the love and security of her home, her marriage, and her family. In this way, she cultivated her yang while nourishing her yin and came closer to her own wholeness.

Moving Beyond the Limits of Duality

One hundred years ago, Jung's hypothesis about the anima and animus was radical, even revolutionary, within the conservative Protestant Swiss culture he was born into. The idea that a man has a woman within him who he needs to know and relate to, and a woman has an interior man who she needs to know and relate to, was enough to send shock waves around the Western world. Yet, although Jung's theory was disputed and at times ridiculed, it took root and, throughout the twentieth century, had a significant influence on the development of modern depth psychotherapy, gender theory, and the dismantling of earlier limiting definitions of masculinity and femininity.

Years ago, when I first learned about Jung's theory, it made sense to me. I recognized the archetype that Jung described as the positive animus come alive in me after my divorce, as I reclaimed certain yang qualities such as assertiveness, penetrating thought, and authoritative confidence that I had projected onto my successful doctor husband. I still feel the influence of the inner partner as I strive to reconcile my desire for intimacy and connection with my ambition and healthy aggression; to balance my emotional vulnerability with my need for freedom, independence, and adventure; and to integrate my yin receptivity with the clear and authoritative expression of my ideas.

In addition, I recognized the archetypes Jung called the negative anima and animus. I had seen them in action as an "unconscious couple" in my marriage when, possessed by my animus or unconscious "other lover," I snapped resentfully at my husband for his lack of empathy instead of clearly articulating my need for deeper relatedness, or when he ran off with his anima, his "other lover," who took the form of endless important conferences, trainings, and work-shops that took precedence over our relatedness. I also lived with the negative expression of anima and animus throughout my childhood in the presence of a highly intelligent, yet non-actualized mother and a sensitive, artistic, yet uncommunicative father who would go at each other in unconscious rounds of bickering and withdrawal. As Jung's theory became real to me, I had no question in my mind that if my mother had been supported in developing her own thinking function and had found a way to express her ideas and use her talents, she would not have resorted to picking and snapping at my father when he returned late from work. And if my father could have valued and listened to his own heart and expressed to my mother what he felt and needed at the level of his soul, he would not have punished her with his contempt and silence, and she would have felt loved and related to.

As I recovered from the earthquake of my divorce, the idea of the positive animus, the "man" who lived within me and who could help me discover my own wholeness, gave me a feeling of support and hopefulness. Gradually, I took my "animus projections" of success, authority, and confident self-expression back from my former hus-band. I came to know those qualities as inborn aspects of my nature, important parts of the wholeness of my Self that had not been rec-ognized or cultivated by my family or culturally endorsed in me as a woman. Eventually, I was able to distinguish between the voice of my authentic inner partner—daring, radical, honest, committed to his values and integrity, available to support my feminine intuition and embodied knowing—with the voice of the negative trickster—snarky, brittle, competitive, self-pitying, victimized, manipulative, and misogynistic. As I entered back into intimate relationships, I felt the support, protection, and discernment of my healthy animus part-ner and could also activate the pause—to wait and not react—when the negative animus tried to take center stage.

Jung's theory of the anima/animus worked well for me. It proved personally useful as I moved out of the safety of my marriage into my life as an independent woman, a single mother, and a pioneer of new ideas about healing. It helped me accept and effectively engage "yang" parts of my own nature that I feared and was confused by. It helped me stop projecting my aggression, ambition, and authority onto men, and instead to own these qualities as complements to my receptivity, sensitivity, and desire for relatedness. On the professional level, the theory helped me unravel relationship problems and life impasses that came up in my work with patients, particularly with people who were relatively well adapted to cultural conventions with regard to their sexual and gender identity.

The theory worked quite well until I met Benjamin and we started to apply these dualistic categories to our own unconventional and uniquely alchemical relationship. In no time, the clear divisions between male and female, anima and animus, dissolved in the quagmire of our gender fluidity and innate queerness—Benjamin's profoundly nurturing nature, his relationality, and well-developed sensate function, with its sustaining and containing capacities, which paradoxically complemented my fiery ambition, initiative, goal orientation, and insatiable drive to understand and articulate my thoughts. On the other hand, at times, Benjamin was the one who demanded we move into new and unchartered territory, who insisted on the positive quality of separation, or withdrew into the yang airy realms of spirit and idealistic visioning. In response, I would transform into the yin partner who called him down to the soul realm of emotion, embodiment, process, and relationality. Within the first weeks of knowing each other, we realized that if we were going to stay in each other's lives, we had to accept that the "he" and "she" as well as the "inner partners" and unconscious couples in our relationship were mutable qualities that shape-shifted moment to moment depending on our growing edges and life challenges. The more we worked with this reality, the more we came to understand that we were not alone in our inability to fit neatly into simple gender-defined binary categories.

As soon as we began teaching anima/animus theory to young people living at the gender-bending closing of the twentieth century, eyes glazed over and disputes broke out. Our students promptly rejected any rigidly defined categories of gender attributes and even questioned the idea that anatomy, hormones, and chromosomal makeup have anything to do with personality development or identity. Same-sex couples felt that the theory did not apply to them and people who were not currently in relationship felt like damaged goods with no hope of psychological redemption. We empathized with their objections, yet still felt strongly that the theory has merit when dealing with psycho-emotional development and healing.

We eventually came to realize that the theory of the anima/animus is a good beginning but it's only half, or maybe just a fraction, of the whole story. The dualistic view of the heterosexual couple as an outer expression of the divine marriage and the completion of psychological wholeness has collapsed in the face of a newly emerging integral consciousness. This new consciousness, which among other things is reshaping our notion of gender and sexual identity, requires a more fluid, dynamic, and holistic model of the Self.

As we sat with the question of where to go from there, I remembered the paradox of cinnabar. I realized that, once again, ancient alchemists were way ahead of their time.

Cinnabar

A Chinese character sometimes used to refer to alchemy is *tan*, which is said to represent a speck of metal being heated in a smelting furnace. The Chinese use the same character to refer to the metal cinnabar, the most prized mineral substance in all of Taoist alchemy. Cinnabar, or mercuric sulfide, is formed through the combining of mercury and sulfur. In alchemical traditions throughout the world, these two metals have come to represent the cosmic principals of yin and yang. Sulfur, which is volatile, hot, and dry, embodies the qualities of yang fire. Mercury, which is silver, cool, and reflective, embodies the qualities of yin water. Sulfur is solar while mercury is lunar. Together, the two reflect the sun and the moon in the form of organic compounds. The composite metal, cinnabar, thus symbolizes the coniunctio, the alchemical marriage of sun and moon, yang and yin, masculine and feminine, which gives rise to the birth to a divine child, the creation of a new wholeness or a new possibility.

But it is the paradox of cinnabar that offers a clue to the deeper meaning of the alchemical marriage. Whereas the shimmery, fluid nature of mercury does reflect qualities we recognize as yin, mercury's surprising and ever-shifting form is also reminiscent of the ejaculation containing male sexual essences and the pure, unfettered consciousness of the spirit. Mercury is the mineral embodiment of yin within yang, the cosmic principal that endows a man with an inner power, enduring sexual potency, and the capacity to not only initiate and impregnate but also to sustain the process of reproduction through his caring for the feminine.

Sulfur embodies the hot, fiery, combustible nature of the yang, but its dark crimson color is reminiscent of menstrual blood and its dense weight and stable form has the feel of matter, heavy flesh, and the physical body. Sulfur is archetypally related to the mysterious darkness of the underworld, the domain of crystals and steaming geysers that spring up from the depths of the earth. Sulfur expresses in mineral form the yang within the yin, the cosmic principal that endows a woman with fertility as well as the capacity to gestate and nourish embryos and eggs and then ride the wild waves of labor that lead to the birth of new life.

The inner opposites hidden in mercury and sulfur contain the secret soul nature of the metals. They are like the dots or eyes of the fish of the Taiji that transform the symbol from a static duality into a dynamic and generative quaternity. They offer us a clue to the alchemy of gender that can help us heal from the painful separations of mental consciousness and discover a new, more integral wholeness within ourselves.

A Four-Part Model of Gender

Creation myths throughout space and time describe the beginning of the universe as a state of primal chaos. A unity, a fertile void, a pure, formless potentiality, an unbroken wholeness the ancient Chinese called *Tao*. This is the state each of us is conceived in and to which we ultimately return. In this time before and after time as we know it, there are no opposites. All exists in Oneness. In Plato's *Symposium*, he has Aristophanes tell a myth that describes people as spherical creatures, round as a globe, with two bodies attached back to back. There were the male-male people, and the female-female people, but there were also male-female people, the androgynous ones. These sphere people tried to take over the gods, so Zeus cut them all in half—the Oneness broken—leaving the navel as a reminder to not defy the gods again.

As I discussed in Chapter 2, the Taoist sage Fu Hsi built an entire philosophy around Tao and the pivotal creation moment when the unknowable Unity divided, bringing the two fundamental opposing cosmic principles of creation into existence. To review, Fu Hsi named these principles *ch'ien*—the yang, creative power of spirit—and *k'un*—the yin, receptive power of matter. In the I Ching, he expressed these principals in the form of simple trigrams—three unbroken lines to represent pure yang and three broken lines to represent pure yin—and placed them on a vertical axis:

Ch'ien - Heaven

K'un - Earth

But then, going further, Fu Hsi added two more trigrams to show how these pure, absolute principles changed as they moved into relative time, space, and embodied form where nothing is pure and absolute. He called the relative expressions of cosmic energy *li*—the yang principal of fire, radiance, east, and the rising sun of morning—and *k'an*—the yin principal of water, darkness, west, and the approaching night.

　　　　　　　　　　　The Alchemy of Inner Work

Fire—li—is yang, active, hot, and bright but there is a blue darkness at its center where it clings to the yin for its sustenance. This paradox of embodiment is represented in the trigram by a broken line that is yin in between the two yang lines.

Water—k'an—is yin, receptive, cool, and dark, but from its depths it reflects the light and power of the sun. This paradox of embodiment is represented in the trigram by a solid line that is yang in between the two yin lines.

Fu Hsi placed the second set of trigrams on a horizontal line perpendicular to the first vertical line.

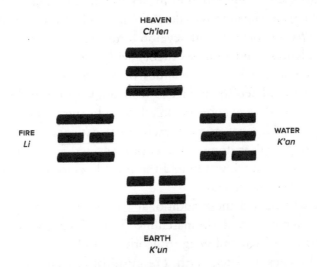

Figure 11. The Four Primary Trigrams

The vertical line represents the formless, infinite, and unchanging realm of spirit. The horizontal line represents the finite world of embodied matter where form is in flux and the only constant is change. The point of confluence between the two lines is the zone where alchemy begins.

Five thousand years after Fu Hsi developed his trigram model of the cosmos, C. G. Jung recognized that the archetype of the syzygy represented this same dynamic in the human psyche. Just as yin water glows at the center of yang fire and yang fire is reflected from the depths of water, Jung had the radical insight that allowed him to see that the feminine nourishes, roots, and completes the masculine while the masculine principle illuminates, activates, and completes the feminine. But less than fifty years after Jung first presented his ideas on the anima and the animus, the theory began to break down in the face of new developments in psychology, the sexual revolution of the 1960s, feminism, gay liberation, the men's movement, and, more recently, the emergence of genderqueer expression within the culture. Other explorers of the psyche, notably theologian and psychologist Genia Pauli Haddon in her groundbreaking book *Uniting Sex, Self & Spirit*, began to reevaluate Jung's work, critique its dualistic, limiting patriarchal bias and develop it further.

As Haddon studied Jung's theory within the context of her own experience and the deeper realities of human sexual anatomy and desire, she modified the model to resonate with the reality of contemporary modern experience. In addition to anima and animus, she found two additional primary archetypal patterns associated with aspects of sexual anatomy—the containing testes and the exertive womb—to which we would add the erectile clitoris in women and the receptive anus in men.

Haddon named these additional biological/psychic archetypes the yang feminine and yin masculine. While Jung assigned the primary pairing of yin and yang to gender as well as unchanging cosmic archetypes—matter, earth, ocean/spirit, heaven, sky—Haddon related the secondary pairing to dynamic change agents. The yin masculine is expressed in the patient holding capacity, the potentiality, and the gathering willpower of the emergent sperm within the testes, while the yang feminine is most clearly seen in the power of the emergent moment, the transformative underworld fire that explodes upward in volcanic eruptions or the propulsive uterine force of labor contractions and the exertive womb at birth.

When we combine the secondary dynamic pair with the primary stable one, the four together form an androgynous symbolic model of basic biological, anatomical, psychic, and cosmic function. Most importantly, we recognize that these four principals are present *in all people, male and female alike.* The four patterns are present in varying degrees of dominance and latency, depending on a multitude of factors that influence any individual life. Healthy and balanced people recognize and relate to all four of these energetic tendencies within themselves and can access them as needed in appropriate response to the inner and outer environment.

This four-part model contains the ancient paradox of Fu Hsi's trigrams as well as the mysterious wholeness of cinnabar. This is our pathway back to our Origin in Tao. It also gives us a clue to the new dynamic, holistic Self structure we need as we move forward into integral consciousness.

Masculinity and Femininity within Yin and Yang
based on the work of Genia Pauli Haddon

Masculine: as it manifests in a man's ego
or in a woman's animus

Feminine: as it manifests in a woman's ego
or in a man's animus

yin-masculine
testicles—self generating/source

developed/optimum:	overdeveloped/exaggerated:	underdeveloped/atrophied:
effective development	procrastination	impatience
resourcefulness	inertia	instability
patience	stagnation	testiness
steadfastness	festering	lack of conviction
abiding presence	stupor	vacuousness
supportive base	sentimentality	fickleness

yang-masculine
phallus—
expanding/penetrating

developed/optimum:

effective development
resourcefulness
patience
steadfastness
abiding presence
supportive base

overdeveloped/exaggerated:

coercive
argumentative
intrusive
rigid
punitive
judgmental

underdeveloped/atrophied:

aimlessness
indecisiveness
fear of going forth
lack of discrimination

yin-feminine
gestative womb—
receiving & incubating

developed/optimum:

nurturing
enclosive
receptive
gestative
inclusive

overdeveloped/exaggerated:

devouring
stifling
overprotective
smothering

underdeveloped/atrophied:

cold
aloof
closed off
inpenetrable

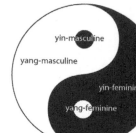

yang-feminine
exertive—pushing & birthing

developed/optimum:	overdeveloped/exaggerated:	underdeveloped/atrophied:
organic transformation	forcing	fearful of change
moving with transformation	refusing	grasping for security
pushing rooted in context	meddling	holding back
intrinsic timing	premature timing	going past term
birthing	aborting	hesitating
developing	abandoning	missing the wave
initiating growth	rejecting	
urging toward completion		

Figure 12. The Four-Part *Yin Yang*

The Alchemy of Inner Work

Chapter 13

Treasuring Darkness

There is no new creation that endures without its concomitant disorder.

   Yet it is the undervaluation of disorder, generally regarded as a state to be escaped at all costs, that is a hallmark of modernity, and rules our historical time.

—Nathan Schwartz-Salant, *The Order-Disorder Paradox*

In the chaos of difficulty at the beginning, order is already implicit.
—The I Ching, Hexagram 3, Difficulty at the Beginning

Diving into the Depths

Many of my patients come to my office at times of crisis. Rachel came just as her mother was dying and her nineteen-year-old college athlete son was experiencing strange bouts of fatigue and weight loss. Rachel described herself as being in the middle of "a perfect storm." And indeed, the storm got worse three months later, when her mother passed away two weeks before her son was diagnosed with cancer.

She was already sobbing in the waiting room when I opened the door to my office. I took her in my arms and held her. When I stepped back and looked in her eyes, I saw dark oceans, uncharted depths, two tunnels without end leading nowhere.

"It's too much," she said. "How does any human being hold all this?"

Inside, I felt the impossibility of words. I said nothing but led her into the office and had her lie down on the treatment table. I held her wrist in my hands. Taking her pulses was like touching rain as it falls into a pond. So many tears—too many tears to count.

In the presence of Rachel's suffering, any order or meaning I could attempt to bring to her experience would be an assault, an insult to the dissolving, disordering magnitude of her experience.

So, what could I do? What can any of us say or do at moments like this, when there is nothing left but not knowing?

Alchemy counsels us to wait and do nothing. Alchemy calls us to go deeper than we believed we could go, to surrender to the currents of life, death, and rebirth, to treasure the lead of embodiment even when the pain is too great to bear, to trust that even when we cannot see, even when we have no answers, and even when all the questions themselves are erased, to hold on to the belief that there is a glint of gold waiting somewhere in the darkness.

Sometimes this is all I can offer my patients—to create with them a space where their healing process can be carried like an embryo, a fetus, a nearly invisible gossamer thread of possibility.

"There's no way for you to hold this," I said. "It's too much for anyone to hold. So, for now, do nothing. Lean back. Feel the table beneath you, the air on your skin. It's enough right now to simply breathe."

Healing the Soul of Our Time

A mother's encounter with her child's death annihilates our human ideas about right order, goodness, or meaning. Yet, Rachel's experience, overwhelming and beyond comprehension as it is, does not feel foreign to me. While her loss is deeply and tragically personal, I also experience it as something familiar, universal. I know in my bones that Rachel's grief is also the grief of the world. If I allow myself to feel the reality of the current moment, I realize that, like Rachel, we are all facing a mind-numbing loss. We are all living in crisis.

As the polar ice caps melt before our eyes, as each year fewer bees and butterflies arrive in our gardens, as the last remaining two thousand-year-old redwood trees succumb to disease, as dozens of species disappear into the void each day, as farmlands dry, forest fires rage, sea levels rise, carcinogens proliferate, and the numbers of homeless refugees swell to unimaginable proportions, we are experiencing the death of the world as we know it. While we attempt to find a place to stand, the ground we have stood upon as a species for the past two hundred thousand years dissolves beneath our feet. As we seek refuge in nature, the very environment that our bodies and nervous systems were designed to inhabit in a synergistic relationship of interbeing is fragmenting. The magnitude of the problem grows greater each day and floods our human capacity for reason, empathy, faith, or grace.

As I approach the closing of this book about modern-day alchemy and healing at this time on our planet, I am daunted by the overwhelming enormity of the lead, the vastness of the illness, the complexity of the systemic disease. But I am also reminded of the numerous ancient alchemical engravings that portray devastated landscapes and shattered vessels. Beside richly colored paintings of celestial weddings, we find images of burning cities charred to smoking ruins, bloodthirsty lions devouring the sun, couples attacking each other tooth and claw, kings beheaded and thrown to dogs. These images point to an alchemical understanding of the primal spiritual necessity for the soul to face and somehow deal with the inevitability of dissolution and death. On the other side of the bleak destruction, there is always moonlight shining when the sunlight dims, green seeds sprouting from the blackened ground, and the rose, always the rose, blossoming alongside the thorns.

And it is here, in this paradox, in the ancient alchemical treasuring of chaos and dissolution, that I find hope. It is in this dismembering fragmentation of meaning that I remember. Anything truly new requires that we somehow find a way to bear the destruction of the old. Without lead, there can be no gold. The miracle of healing transcends my ego's capacity to predict or understand. And it is into this ocean of mystery that I must be willing to swim if I am to truly enter the laboratory and move forward with the work at hand.

Nigredo

Nigredo, as I've defined before, means "darkening." In alchemy, the nigredo is the contracting complement to the coniunctio's bright expansion. Like yin and yang, the coniunctio and nigredo engender each other. With every marriage, every birth, every heart-opening connection, an opposing force of shadow and separation simultaneously arises.

At the closing of every workshop that I lead, I remind participants that there will likely be a let-down, a feeling of abandonment and aloneness afterward. The more powerful the connections that happen and the insights that arise during our time together, the more destabilizing the disorder that may follow. I've found that it's especially important for me to be careful when driving home after I've done a strong piece of work with a group of students as cars appear out of nowhere, deer leap from the side of the highway, or I end up taking wrong exits that leave me stranded on one-way streets. I've also observed that Benjamin and I have had some of our most memorable knock-down, drag-out fights after we've wrapped up a great weekend of inspired teaching. At this point, I accept that a nigredo will follow any expansive growth experience. It's best for me to be prepared for it, care for it, and welcome it as an aspect of the integration process.

In fairy tales, the nigredo is represented by the uninvited thirteenth fairy who shows up with a curse at the celebratory feast of the newborn princess. In the creative process, it is the debilitating self-doubt and critical voices that attack us after a time of rich productivity. In new love, it is the first argument. It is post-partum depression, the setting of the sun, the waning of the full moon, the tipping back down of the sheng cycle at the height of Summer.

Governed by the laws of entropy, mortality, and time, the nigredo represents the resistance of yang spirit to its earthly fall. It is our inevitable encounter with the downward pull of gravity, with the restricting limits of time and space and the inevitability of disintegration. The nigredo is a reality that cannot be eradicated, but with consciousness it can be worked with. Through our conscious acceptance of the nigredo and our willingness to bear its slow and painful wearing down of illusion, the light of spirit incarnates to illuminate the flesh of the soul. As we learn to hold steady through the pride-shredding ordeals, despairs, rages, and initiatory suffering of the nigredo, our sense of Self is strengthened. As we pass through the nigredo, our insights and ideas gather weight and take root in the form of action in our everyday life, our relationships grow through enduring the trials of separation and doubt. In this way, we benefit and are guided by the underworld wisdom of the night.

Black

At the root of alchemy is the power of blackness. Returning to the etymology I discussed in Chapter 1, even our modern English word *alchemy* is infused with *kem*—the root Egyptian word for the rich, black earth and the fertility of the dark soil of the Nile valley. In addition, kem suggests the black color of lead and other metal ores hidden underground.

Kem also had another more esoteric meaning for the Egyptians. The word was used to refer to the shining blackness of the pupil at the center of the eye. The kem of the pupil contains a special kind of blackness that is associated not only with its capacity to absorb and transform light into images but also with its ability to act as a tiny mirror that reflects back in miniature the images of the outer world. This reflective capacity of the pupil is especially activated in the presence of the lover who gazes into the eye of the beloved. In his essay *The Perfect Black*, alchemist and scholar Aaron Cheak writes:

> On one hand, just as the moon is the receiver and reflector
> of the sun's light, so too is the pupil of the eye the feminine,
> receptive function of the solar eye. At the same time however,
> it must be recognized that the feminine aspect of the divine eye
> also had an active function alongside its passive or receptive
> role. The feminine aspect of the divine eye played a crucial role
> . . . she is the *medium* through which the masculine principle

engenders itself . . . the "Mistress of the Universe" . . . the rearing cobra that appeared on the crowns of the Pharaohs.

For the Egyptians, blackness symbolized divine power made manifest. Furthermore, they understood that power comes not only from the masculine principal of the heavens above but also and equally from the feminine principal of the Earth below. In their myths, the light at the center of Horus's eye was given to him by his mother Isis. The power of sight of the sky-god was a gift he received from the Divine Feminine.

The Nekyia or Night Sea Journey

Throughout this book, I've emphasized that the ultimate goal of alchemical work is the activation of the shen from its burial place in the matrix of matter and the body. Taoist alchemists referred to this work as the blossoming of the Golden Flower and European alchemists spoke of it as the discovery of the Philosopher's Stone. From an alchemical perspective, the light of the gold you seek does not shine down from above, but rather rises up from the darkness below. Inner radiance and illuminated sight emerge only after you have sacrificed the knowing brightness of the ego.

The quickening of the shen is most often precipitated by something we would never choose, by the opposite of what we recognize as grace or blessing. It often begins with a shock that disrupts our notion of cause and effect, thrusting us into a confusing chaos, a fathomless void. It began for Rachel when she learned of her son's diagnosis and continued on after his death when she fell, like Sleeping Beauty, into a paralyzing inertia that lasted for several years.

The *Nekyia* or night sea journey is a mythological motif, an archetype, that symbolically describes the nigredo phase of the alchemical process. The Nekyia takes you on a nocturnal voyage. You are swallowed by whales, left to wander in murky marshlands and become entrapped in enchanted forests. One of the earliest versions of the Nekyia comes from ancient Egypt, where the sun god Re drowns and dies each night in the primeval oceanic depths of the water god Nun and is reborn each morning with the sunrise. In Sumeria, the goddess

Inanna willingly descends to the realm of Ereshkigal, the Queen of Death, in order to be initiated and claim her full powers. In Greece, Persephone is abducted to the Underworld by Hades and Odysseus's ocean voyage takes him away from home for most of his adult life.

The motif of the Nekyia is found in ancient stories and legends, but it is also found in the here and now through the experiences of our lives. The Nekyia is happening each day to each of us, in real time. Birth and death are night sea journeys as is sleep. All healing processes that lead to greater integrity and wholeness require a Nekyia of some kind. Inner work that leads to the integration of a disowned part of the Self will bring you through the dismembering and resurrecting energies of this realm. It is the journey each of us is facing now as, for the first time in the history of our species, we've been presented with the prospect of our own extinction as a result of climactic or nuclear catastrophe.

The paradox of the Nekyia is that its chaos both destroys and creates. The descent is the turning point, the critical moment when you at last are forced to let go and surrender, when all the outmoded structures of your life dissolve and new possibilities are born. Rather than resist it or deny that it's happening, regard it as a necessary part of your soul's development and honor its power. Through bearing its loss, you gain. If you survive the trial, like Vasilisa, who survives her encounter with the legendary Russian witch Baba Yaga, you return with a gift—an inner fire that allows you to see in the darkness.

The Mysterious Pass

After many years of studying the Five Element Wheel, I discovered that it has embedded within it a graphic representation of a Nekyia. It is a map that can help us navigate the night sea journey as well as the chaos of our age. Circling the Wheel from Water to Wood to Fire to Earth to Metal, we trace the circular unfolding of the organic processes of carbon-based life—elemental, vegetative, and biological change in our time-bound world.

At the close of Winter, Water rises through the stems of plants to support the growth and negentropic directionality of Wood in Spring.

Wood burns to feed the expansive light and heat of the Fire that defines Summer.

Fire fuels the generative processes of organic matter that produce the generous nourishing abundance of Earth in late Summer.

Finally, Earth disintegrates to form compost and the buried crystalline mineral structures of Metal in the Autumn season.

But then we arrive at a riddle.

How do the inert crystals and minerals of Metal rise again as the vital life-giving power of Water? How is the life force resurrected from the most entropic point of the cycle back to potent negentropy? What is it that reinvigorates the Wheel of Life and allows it to continue to turn on and on through time without running down?

When I was in acupuncture school asking these questions, my teachers never offered satisfactory explanations. Over many years of personal research into myths, symbols, etymology, and perhaps most importantly, observation of the universal qualities inherent to the healing processes of my patients, I finally put the pieces together. The answers to these questions reside at the bottom of the Wheel, in what I have come to call the Mysterious Pass, where Metal is buried and then reborn as vital, potentized Water.

At this point in the process, change does not follow the orderly, rhythmic alternation of night and day, or the predictable cycles of the Elements and the Seasons, or the linear stages of organic growth. The change that happens between Metal and Water is archaic, primal, fundamental. It is a leap or mutation invisible to ordinary sight. It is a radical interruption of a natural cycle that happens outside of ordinary time, akin to labor contractions, earthquakes, hurricanes, or the descriptions we read of near-death experiences, when our usual ways of orienting to the world dissolve and we approach the zero point that lies between being and nonbeing. This is the point of discontinuity where the unfolding of organic process breaks down. At the very bottom of the Wheel is the place of a miracle, where *wu xing*—the world of matter—is penetrated and reinvigorated by the potent spiritual energies of the unseen Underworld.

What I've come to understand is that at the bottom, in this shadow realm at the most yin point of the Wheel, between the

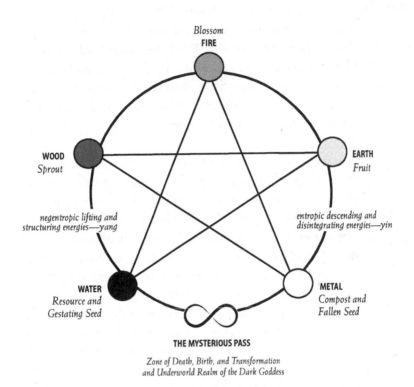

Blossom
FIRE

WOOD
Sprout

EARTH
Fruit

*negentropic lifting and
structuring energies—yang*

*entropic descending and
disintegrating energies—yin*

WATER
*Resource and
Gestating Seed*

METAL
*Compost and
Fallen Seed*

THE MYSTERIOUS PASS

*Zone of Death, Birth, and Transformation
and Underworld Realm of the Dark Goddess*

Figure 13. The Mysterious Pass

alchemical Elements of Metal and Water, we discover a doorway to the cavern of the Dark Goddess. The Mysterious Pass is the domain of *Xi Wang Mu*, the Queen Mother of the West, the Taoist mythological Goddess of Life, Death, and Rebirth, where spirit incarnates and inert matter comes back to life. Here is where we are invited to let go, to surrender, to exhale into the emptiness and trust that the divine will be there to carry us through to our next inhalation.

In this darkness, in the place where we truly cannot see and where our rational mind is rendered powerless, something is coming to life. In this chaos of new beginnings, there is already an implicit form. In the lead of impasse, death, and destruction, there is already the promise of a hidden spark of gold. Dennis William Hauck offers this elegant insight into the alchemical mystery of this place of opacity, lead, and darkness as it relates to our own healing:

Even the elemental metal carries the seed of its own redemption. The alchemists knew that Fire is lord over lead, for the metal has a low melting point and is easily separated from its ore by roasting in an open flame, and the metal itself melts in a candle flame. Lead expands on heating and contracts on cooling more than any other solid heavy metal.

. . . lead carries deeply hidden within its structure the fire of its own transformation. Many lead salts reveal a whole rainbow of brilliant colors, with the solar colors of yellow, orange, and red predominating. This is why lead has been used in paints for so many centuries. Finely divided lead powder is pyrophoric ("fire containing") and easily catches fire or erupts spontaneously in flames. When made into a fine powder, lead metal must be kept in a vacuum to keep from catching fire. Otherwise, it ignites and burns down to a bright yellow ash, revealing its deeply hidden solar signature. So, the wonder of lead is that hidden deep inside the gray, dead metal is a tiny, eternal spark that is the seed of its own resurrection. In the eyes of alchemists, this makes lead the most important metal despite its unattractive darkness. For dull lead and gleaming gold are really the same things, only at different stages of growth or maturity.

The Secret Fire inside lead is really the alchemical basis for transforming lead into gold, and correspondingly, gives mankind hope for its own spiritual transformation. That tiny spark of light in the darkest part of matter makes resurrection part of the structure of the universe.

It is our task to have faith that we can pass through this Grand Darkness to be reborn on the other side, that we can be obliterated without perishing. This faith is the gift of alchemy. We have the map as well as the keys to the laboratory. The Dark Goddess is waiting for us to open the door.

The Dark Goddess

Xi Wang Mu, Queen Mother of the Western Paradise, Most Honored One, Empress of the Immortals, the most ancient and revered of all the Taoist deities, presides over the realm of Birth, Life, Death, and Resurrection. She represents the spiritual principle of matter, the power of the yang feminine. She is the potency of the uterus, the will of the seed, the high-grade energy sequestered in the oil reserves, the negentropic upward thrust of geysers and hot springs. She oversees all organic processes, from the slow disintegration of stones to the ephemeral life of a luna moth to the gestation, birth, growth, and decay of a tree, a mountain, a flowing river, of your own bones and body.

The Queen lives far beyond the reach of the conscious mind, deep in the caves below the sacred Kunlun Mountain of China. Her mountain is inhabited by fantastical beings and shamanistic emissaries. Among them are the three-footed crow, the nine-tailed fox, a dancing frog, and the moon-hare who pounds minerals, mixes herbs, and prepares her magical elixirs in a mortar. There are phoenixes and dancing maidens and azure lads, and spirits riding on white stags. She resides here, in this place that is infinitely deep, infinitely dark. A place with no beginning and no end, in a body that also has no beginning and no end.

In the ancient texts, the Queen is described as a fearsome creature with a human face, tiger's teeth, and a leopard's tail, wild hair flowing about her as she sits on the three-legged stool that is her throne, above the yellow sulfur springs of the Underworld. At the center of her palace on Kunlun Mountain is a magic fountain where the Feast of the Immortals takes place. Her meats include bear paws, monkey lips, and dragon livers; for dessert, she dines on the peach of immortality that ripens every three thousand years from her magic tree.

She, like all her other fearsome sisters—Ereshkigal, the Sumerian Lady of the Great Place Below; Pele, the Hawaiian Goddess of Volcanoes; Baba Yaga, the Russian Witch of the Forest—walks through flames without ever getting burned, has a voracious appetite, a nasty sense of humor, and zero tolerance for fools. And yet, at other times, the Queen Mother is described as a compassionate, exquisite, and gracious goddess who presides over the Peach Orchards of Immortality and endows her visitors with health, renewal, and even everlasting life.

What is the magic, what is the incantation, what is the prayer, that transforms the ravenous monster of the Underworld into the gracious goddess of orchards and fountains? And how many more years will it take for her peaches to once again ripen on the branches of her sacred tree?

Severed in two by the separating mind of mental consciousness throughout the past five hundred years, Xi Wang Mu has lived a dual life. Subdued by the patriarchal gods and the kings of medieval China, one part of the Goddess sits demurely on an alabaster throne dressed in courtly, silken gowns as she falls in love with mortals and sings to her pet birds. This aspect of the Goddess became a paragon of female skill, grace, and beauty for medieval Chinese poets and painters. Today, with the extreme secularization and materialization in the People's Republic of China, she has all but disappeared from view.

But another part of Xi Wang Mu lives on in China as well as in the collective unconscious of humanity. Dishonored and relegated to the shadow, this other aspect of the Goddess becomes the Night Mare, the hysteric, the Thirteenth Fairy who shows up to cast the death spell at our feast of life. Darkness has become the enemy rather than the partner of Light. Matter has become a tomb of annihilation rather than a womb of gestation. The body and all of Nature an unwieldy machine we endlessly try to fix and control. Feelings of foreboding, anxiety, and terror combined with compulsive activity and the desperate attempt to impose order on the world eclipse our creative capacities for introspection, surrender, rest, renewal, and the surprising new possibilities that arise in the presence of her deep Underworld wisdom.

When consciousness is overly dominated by phallocentric mental attitudes, reverence for the darkness, the night, myths and dreams, and the spacious wandering of the unconscious are no longer valued as necessary aspects of a spiritually balanced life. Rather, in the face of the ultimate power of the yin, of entropy, death, and darkness, our modern consciousness responds with adrenal-fueled activity, denial, and an exhausting, futile attempt to outrun her relentless tidal pull.

If we shift our view and approach the Goddess's dark depths with respect and compassion, we can begin to receive the benefit of her support and wisdom. Whenever we face a life-threatening disease or come to terms with the process of aging, any time we're brought to our knees by loss, addiction, or pain, she is waiting to receive us into her infinite mystery. When we reach an impasse in our work life, our relationships, our creativity, we can choose to surrender to the unknown, to reverse the handle of the stars and turn inward, following the thread that leads us back to our own source . . . to the Self, to the Tao.

Over the long months and years that I sat with Rachel after her son's death, she and I often sat in silence. Infinities passed between our words. At moments, I felt myself reduced to a transparent body without voice or substance in the face of her annihilating despair. The one certainty I had was that there was nothing I could say or do to make things better for her.

When I treated Rachel with needles or essential oils, the only way I stayed fully present to the pain was by simultaneously channeling healing energy to my own heart, reminding my feet to reach down to receive the sustaining energies of the Earth. In order to hold the space for Rachel's devastation, I had to continually regulate and calm the shock waves that rocked through my own nervous system in the presence of hers. The one thing that sustained me, the only thing I knew, was to turn this suffering over to the Dark Goddess.

And so, week after week, again and again, I would lean back into her night black skirts. I would swim out into her wide, devouring ocean. Silently, but with all my strength, I would call on the Goddess to support me through this session and the next. Behind me, I could feel her wide, inscrutable eyes opening a gateway back to origin. I would take a breath and lean back further. Then the wind would shift, and I could feel her there in the room. With Rachel. With me. With all of us here on the planet, struggling to heal a wound too great to feel, to stay present to life and death in the same moment.

Revisioning Death

As a healer, I have watched death. I have watched people die and I have witnessed people watch others die. I watched as one of my patients fought multiple myeloma for fifteen years before he died, spending millions of dollars to fight tooth and nail to the very last days. I watched as my wild older brother went out in a blaze of glory, never admitting he had Stage 4 lung cancer until a few days before he succumbed, swiftly and with very little fuss, as he preferred, saying simply and without fanfare, "I'm leaving now."

I've come to realize that there are an infinite variety of ways to die. There are deaths that are sweet and timely, like my mother's. There are deaths that rip your heart from your body and tear it into a thousand ragged pieces, like Rachel's son's. And there are deaths that come too late, like the death of a friend who spent her final decade waiting in a nursing home for something she could no longer name or remember.

What I have come to understand through watching death is that it is not the enemy. Although there are times when it is very wrong and times when it is absolutely right, death is not the problem our culture makes it out to be. Just as our lack of reverence for the Dark Goddess has turned her into a fearsome Bitch Goddess, it is our attitude toward death that has turned it into a devouring monster. Fighting this monster, somehow postponing or arresting the entropic power of its yin mystery, has become the final, and ultimately futile, battle of patriarchal mental consciousness. As a central component of this full-scale war, fighting death and prolonging the life span has become the obsession of our modern health care system. This focus, while benefitting investors in the pharmaceutical, insurance, medical research, and technology sectors, is draining vast stores of time, money, and intellectual resources that could be used to promote planetary well-being, including care for the young and underserved, preventive health initiatives, and detoxification of the environment.

Death has become such a horrifying beast in our culture that it's nearly taboo to talk about it. On many occasions, Rachel told me that she noticed friends avoiding her when she went shopping or walked along the path by the river. "They look away," she'd report, "or, when

The Alchemy of Inner Work

we meet, they talk about themselves and act like nothing's happened or, worst of all, they ask if I'm feeling better." This awkwardness and lack of honoring rituals in our culture reflects an attempt to deny the ultimate power of the Dark Goddess. The tragedy is that this denial is not only futile, it also robs us of the benefits of death's redemptive power and its necessary lessons for the soul.

One of the most important understandings I've received from the wisdom world of alchemy is that death is a part of life. The two are not separate. When we resist the nigredo, the death phase, whether in a relationship, a project, or a life, we are also resisting the powerful energies of renewal. The Dark Goddess destroys what needs to die in order for life to continue. There are, of course, deaths where this is easier to accept than others. There are deaths of marriages that, while sad, unleash an abundance of creativity and eros. There are deaths of illusions and infatuations that open the door for freedom and growth. And there are deaths of elders that make way for younger, more vital energies.

And then there are situations, like Rachel's, where this alchemical principle crashes against a rock-hard wall and hits a "no" that shakes the foundation of our cosmos. There are situations, like the perilous deaths of leopards, gorillas, and sea turtles—all species at risk of extinction, the death of the coral reefs, the deaths worldwide of millions of people each year from hunger. How do we honor the Dark Goddess when she annihilates what we love?

Returning Current

After a time of decay comes the turning point. The powerful light that has been banished returns. There is movement but it is not brought about by force.

—The I Ching, Hexagram 24, Return

For years after her son's death, Rachel continued to feel numb and hopeless. There were moments when I thought I should be doing more, trying harder, giving some kind of helpful advice. Another part of me trusted that the task I had been given through our work together was to bear witness to her suffering, to hold steady and not be overwhelmed by her grief, to put my hands on her feet, to remind her that she still lived in a body.

Then, for a while, she stopped coming. I thought of calling to check in but decided against it. I decided to wait and see what happened.

When she returned, something was different. There in the dark tunnel of her gaze, I saw a tiny spark and I knew she was *seeing* me, clearly, perhaps for the first time. There had been a dream. Her son was little, and she was putting him to bed. She covered him carefully with a blanket and sang him to sleep. When she woke up, she knew that after years of resistance, it was time for her to let go of the ashes she kept in a box in her son's bedroom. It was time to take them to the river and let them go.

She watched the dust as it blew like gray pollen in the wind. She watched it settle on the black water and slowly sink below. Then, she said, she felt that there was really nothing left to live for. No, she would never take her life, but she would never fully live again.

But later that same day, as she was working in her garden, digging some weeds that had grown up around a small pile of stones, she felt something in the soil, something not rock or root, but cool and round like a coin. She dug down deeper, clawing the dirt away with her fingernails. She dug around the edges of the object, until she could manage to release it from the grip of the earth that had hardened around it. She pulled it up.

It was a small round disc, a St. Christopher's medal, the patron saint of children and travelers, the very one who carried a child, unknown to him, across a mighty river, a child who later was revealed as Christ.

As a young girl, her mother placed such a medal around her neck for safety and protection, but she had not seen one since. She had no idea where it had come from or how it had made its way into the garden. But she cleaned it up, put it on a chain, and was now wearing it around her neck.

Stories like Rachel's that shake the foundation of what we believe is real and possible happen when we draw close to the realm of death and transformational healing. The shattering grief and the encounter with chaos force us to surrender our fixed ideas about reality. This reorientation is a part of the process of soul-level healing—the realization that we don't know, that we cannot know, and yet something way bigger than our limited ego does know and can, if we listen carefully enough, help us to understand.

In the years I spent working with Rachel and many other patients going through loss and grief, I learned the lesson of limitation. I learned that the only thing I can do in response to the magnitude, the madness, the incomprehensible suffering we face when we come into a body, is do everything I can to remain present.

If I had tried to force some kind of logic onto Rachel's experience or to fix things for her in any way, she would have surely fled. And, if she had not found the fortitude to stay in the work—without hope, without expectation, without demanding that anything change— then the crack in the egg of ordinary time and causal linear reality would not have happened for her. We would have missed the Dark Goddess, would not have felt her brushing us lightly as she passed by. Solutions, if there are to be any for Rachel, or for any of us living at this time of death and rebirth and chaotic transformation on our planet, can only come through letting go of trying to make things work out the way we want them to. The solutions will come from another dimension, another time, through our deep listening. They will only arise from the integrity we cultivate in our relationships to ourselves, with each other, and through our capacity to trust the healing power of love.

Touching the medal around her neck, Rachel looked at me and said, "It's impossible but true. And I guess I have to take it as a message. It's time for me to let him go. He needs to get on with his own journey, as do I."

Alchemy tells us that renewal is possible after illness, after loss, after despair, and even after death, but it can only come through a surrender and a descent into darkness. It cannot be bought, bargained for, or forced through the personal will. Its timing is not under conscious control. The returning current can only be cared for, cultivated, and dreamed into becoming. Just as when, at the still point of Winter, a black line cracks the ice and deep below sleeping seeds stir in their dark beds, so vision and hope return when the conditions and the timing are favorable.

As we face the disintegration of a world that has forgotten that life and death are connected and that darkness is the necessary companion to the light, we must resist the impulse to cling onto familiar thought patterns or to reason our way through to premature, one-sided solutions. Equally, giving in to denial, cynicism, and despair, while tempting, will not serve the renewal of the world. It is crucial not to give up hope. It is crucial to renew our capacity for telepathy and magic. To tell stories and sing songs. And to think clearly when clear thinking is called for.

The medicine needed to support this renewal is a distillation of patience and faith along with a deep and abiding reverence for the power of the Underworld. We must form new tribes and build new laboratories and remind each other, again and again, that if we bring the spirit of love back to the realm of matter, the yin tendency toward entropy will reverse. Then the streams, rivers, and oceans of life will begin to flow again. Fish will return to the waters and birds to the sky, and all manner of fantastic dream creatures will walk easily between our imagination and the natural world. Past and future will embrace in this one ever-present moment and then, as we read in Hexagram 24 of the I Ching, ". . . the transformation of the old becomes easy. The old is discarded and the new is introduced."

Conclusion

A New Story of Healing

Behold! It is the eve of time, the hour when the wanderers turn toward their resting-place. One god after another is coming home. . . . Therefore, be present.

—Jean Gebser, *The Ever-Present Origin*

As you come to the conclusion of this book and turn your attention back to the hyper-kinetic sound bites of our current reality—the endless input of alarming images on television, the negativity of the news, and the fragmented cacophony of cyber tweets and internet reports—the alchemical stories, ideas, and inner practices I have shared may begin to fade like dreams from your awareness. The subtle, twilight realm of alchemy may be quickly overshadowed by the glare of mental consciousness, the demands of everyday life, and the overwhelming magnitude of the challenges facing humanity at the present time.

As the world around us careens toward increasing states of environmental, financial, and cultural chaos, and the time and resources available for poetry, dreaming, self-reflection, imagination, and creativity shrink, does personal healing at a soul level still matter?

How can a young boy's recovery from the trauma of an unexpected chronic illness, a feisty psychotherapist's struggle to find herself without leaving her marriage, a coyote-spirited singer searching for the courage to sing, an advertising executive's development of an inner life, a mother's annihilating experience of her son's death, how can the courageous, creative inner work of these brief individual lives matter in the face of climate change, species extinction, monster storms, disappearing rain forests, endless numbers of homeless and incarcerated people, rampant racism, crumbling democracies, destroyed cultures, and genocides?

After more than three decades spent with patients in the treatment room and two decades spent developing my work with Alchemical Healing, I feel the painful relevance of this question rock through every cell in my body. And yet, the answer that comes from the depth of my heart is, yes, the soul still matters because it is the essence of our humanity.

And yes, one person's resolute audacity to heal, to find meaning and purpose, and to evolve at a soul level does matter because in the integral reality that is struggling to emerge, one person's inner work touches us all. In this new consciousness, our personal growth will inevitably result in some positive, albeit unpredictable, change in the outer world. Indeed, as I learned during the weekend I spent with Joanna Macy, inner work and the consciousness shifts it engenders are prerequisites for healing the planet.

In the latest research on the theory of evolution, the accepted Darwinian idea of natural selection and the survival of the fittest is being re-examined. Ornithologist and evolutionary biologist Richard O. Prum, in his book *The Evolution of Beauty*, proposes that "evolution is frequently far quirkier, stranger, more historically contingent, individualized, and less predictable and generalizable than adaptation can explain." In fact, according to Prum, evolution is guided not only by rational, measurable, predictable survival strategies but also by a mysterious subjectivity and by individual aesthetic experiences of beauty and desire.

In his book *Climate: A New Story*, Charles Eisenstein asks, "What induces a shift to the consciousness of interbeing?" And with an indirect nod to Prum's view of evolution, Eisenstein answers his own question "It is through a confrontation with beauty, suffering, and mortality. It is through a confrontation with what is real."

The innate entelechy of life to grow in the direction of truth, beauty, and wholeness that underlies all of alchemy as well as Prum's thesis and Eisenstein's reply also forms the basis of Alchemical Healing. For me, it also explains why the soul, with its miraculous capacity to reverse entropy and reinvigorate the life force with courage, hope, connection, compassion, and inspiration, still matters, perhaps more now than ever before.

And yet, the caveat is that the zeitgeist of our time requires that Alchemical Healing extend beyond our individual soul's experience of healing and growth if it is to provide a relevant and useful new story of health and healing. Although I am convinced that fulfilling the mandate of our unique Tao is still a crucial aspect of a fully realized life, there is more. We also need to move beyond the myth of the Hero's Journey, the successful fulfillment of individual destiny, which is the central theme of mental consciousness and the Western project. We must discover a life path that includes and goes beyond Jung's individuation process.

We need to find a way to heal and fulfill our destinies as individuals within a tribe and an integrated circle of life, where one person's well-being does not detract from the well-being of the community or come at the expense of harm to other beings or the environment. In her book *Emergent Strategy*, social justice activist and healer Adrienne Maree Brown writes, "Right now, it's clear to me that something is wrong if it hurts the planet." She adds, "We all have the capacity to heal each other—healer is a possibility in each of us." And she asks, "How can we, future ancestors, align ourselves with the most resilient practices of emergence as a species?"

Clearly, a view of healing that takes into account the well-being and destiny of the individual as well as the well-being and destiny of the human community and the planet is the new possibility. And just as clearly, none of us know how to do it yet. We are living in a group learning project, a vast human laboratory experiment with a completely uncertain outcome. In the depths of our being, we feel something attempting to arise, something buried like a seed within us, something that knows and yet, requires a sacrifice of knowing. This not yet manifest but implicit possibility requires us to come out of numbness and denial, to feel our fear, anger, love, generosity, and grief in the face of illness, impasse, crisis, and death. It demands that we revise our view of the body from a problematic mechanical system to a sacred source of wisdom, and that we care for the world as we would for our own body. This new possibility invites us to surrender familiar but no longer efficient ways of organizing our reality in order to give birth to a radically new way of being a healthy human.

Here are some simple questions that could be helpful as we move forward along the uncertain path of our journey—for me, for you, for anyone with the resources to access health care. These are questions without right or wrong answers, in keeping with the ambiguity and rigorous self-reflection that is central to Alchemical Healing. I believe that if we are willing to wrestle with the challenges these questions present, they might help guide us, one decision at a time, toward a more integral and sustainable approach to healing.

How do my decisions about my health affect the natural environment?

Are they in harmony with my time, my age, and my Tao?

Do they make sense in terms of financial costs and returns? Who truly foots the bill? Who benefits?

Am I making a decision about my health care because I am afraid of death or because I truly have more to learn or contribute in this lifetime?

How will this decision benefit my family, my community, and the planet? How will it allow me to give back more?

Looking deeply into the eyes of all the children of all the beings who currently inhabit this miraculous planet, what commitment will I make to their health and wholeness in the future?

If *healing*, *whole*, and *holy* derive from the same root, what does it mean for me to be truly healthy?

There are glimmers here of higher octaves, new frequencies, previously unknown radio stations, expanding dimensions, opening chakras, and reorganizing neurological synapses. The speck of starlight we receive at the moment of our conception is a point, a unique scintilla that guides us in a particular direction, and yet our North Star shines with the infinite light of a multitude of other stars. This is the paradox at the heart of Alchemical Healing as we move forward into the eve of time.

Acknowledgments

Benjamin and I met in May 1996 at a workshop called The Body Sacred where we were exploring the connections between relationships, sex, and spirit. I was a practicing acupuncturist, two years out of a marriage with a holistic physician, a self-identified mystic and feminist. Benjamin was beginning his work as an astrologer, was thirteen years younger than me, and at that time identified as a gay man.

Unexpectedly, by the end of the first evening of the workshop, we found ourselves lying on the floor of the main conference room getting to know each other through the lens of our astrology charts. As different as our lives appeared on the surface, we discovered that in addition to our fascination with the planets and stars, we shared a passionate interest in a wide array of subjects, including spirituality, sexuality, social justice, community, healthy food, and alternative healing. We were both actively engaged in our own healing. Benjamin was recovering from the challenge of growing up as a sensitive, mystical, intellectually curious boy in a large, baseball-obsessed, working-class Catholic family haunted by the ghosts of alcoholism and incest. I was making my peace with the contradictions of my family's impoverished, trauma-filled Rumanian Jewish past and the heady brew of Eastern spirituality, European romanticism, modern art, Madison Avenue advertising, and Hollywood fantasy that infused my upper middle-class suburban childhood.

Nearly ten years later, after a prolonged relationship practice period that included multiple break ups and reconciliations, monogamous and non-monogamous sexual agreements, snail mails and emails, and living for five years on opposite sides of the country, Benjamin and I surrendered to our connection and decided to try living together under one roof. We knew intuitively, as well as from our composite astrology chart, that our life together was going to be about service to others. We also knew that being together as a couple would require that we relinquish conventional ideas about male and female gender roles, about age and power, as well as sexual, class, and cultural identity. We weren't going to have children and we weren't financially dependent on each other. If we were going to be lifelong partners, we would need something besides family, finances, cultural connections, and social status to keep us together. We knew that the "something" would be bigger than just us, that it was related to the "something" that kept bringing us back together no matter how hard we tried to separate. It had to do with how we invited each other to grow even when it hurt and how we never stopped supporting each other's true nature and purpose even when it felt threatening or difficult to understand. It had something to do with the Fire and Air in our respective astrology charts that kept our commitment to healing burning steadily despite many moments of doubt, betrayal, hurt, anger, and despair. It had something to do with our shared longing to be part of the creation of a more peaceful, beautiful, just, and healthy world. Put simply, it had something to do with our souls.

The breakthrough came one rainy weekend. We were visiting our mutual friend, sipping tea and wondering about next steps forward. Benjamin was tired of his work organizing conferences and trainings for a nonprofit and I had reached a standstill in my teaching and clinical practice. He was looking for a way to combine his organizational skills with his passion for astrology and inner work and I was ready to share the tools of Alchemical Healing with a larger audience. Out of the blue, Benjamin sat up. "I got it," he exclaimed. "Everything we do is about helping people figure out how to create new possibilities for themselves. We need to develop that vision. We need a community. We need to find a way to bring people together to discover what it means to be truly healthy. I want to create an organization called A New Possibility."

A few years later, A New Possibility became an entity and we launched our website. We combined Benjamin's vision and organizational expertise with my clinical and teaching experience to cocreate the Alchemical Healing Mentorship, which became the foundational program of our work. In addition to our clinical practices, we now maintain multiple ongoing healing and learning communities, along with online classes and retreat programs, that teach people how to work with the soul to help themselves and others live more healthy, purposeful, and vibrant lives as they consciously contribute to the healing of their communities and the planet.

In 2012, when we finally stood in the rambling field adjacent to our vegetable garden in Maine, witnessed by our community, family, friends, and former lovers, we promised to continue to support the emergence of each other's complicated, unique, and authentic nature in service of healing and wholeness, both in ourselves and on the planet. We knew that there were far more than just the two of us exchanging vows that September day. A plethora of partners join in every marriage, in every creative project undertaken, including the writing of this book.

As we consider the many people who have supported us, we make a final nod to our students, clients, and patients who have been our true alchemical teachers. In addition, we are blessed with such a multitude of friends that it would be impossible to name each one individually, but there are a few who we do need to thank by name. Roger Leggat, you were with us when we met at The Body Sacred. Ever since, you have been unwavering in your generosity and have stayed committed to the precious friendship we have worked to cultivate. Nathan Schwartz-Salant and Lydia Salant, you are irreplaceable! You have taught us about coniunctios and nigredos like nobody's business. Lydia, we still feel you teaching us from the other side. Michael Gelb and Deb Domanski Gelb, your genius astonishes! Thank you for your gracious hospitality, persistent optimism, and bright spirits.

Thank you to our team at Cynthia Cannell Literary Agency— Cynthia Cannell, Charlotte Kelly, and Nico Brown. Cynthia, from our first conversation, you got what I wanted to achieve with this book. Your support has made a world of difference.

A bow of deep gratitude to our editor, Peter Turner, and the entire team at Red Wheel/Weiser. Peter, you are an alchemist par excellence! Not only did you see the gold in the lead of the original four hundred and fifty-page manuscript, but you have offered wise counsel throughout the writing process as we refined our vision and our voice.

Our dear dreamer, stargazer, and gemstone magician, Laura Givertz, you are our companion on this journey and an ever-present inspiration to our souls. Thank you for being willing to read every word of the early drafts. Even when the text was raw and messy, you helped us see the light that was shining through the darkness. Thanks also to George Hurvitt, Sarah Juster, and Jessie Shaw for your support as readers.

Our thanks to others who have been important threads in the weaving of our work. Dr. Rudy Ballentine, our gratitude for the pivotal role you played in lighting the spark. Dr. Kathryn Rensenbrink, friend, colleague, and walking partner, thanks for our inspirational conversations about medicine. Richard Spera, your willingness to share the beauty of your life with us and our students has inspired us to believe more deeply in new possibilities. Erica Moffet, you nourished the body and soul of the Alchemical Healing Mentorship for years before joining the acupuncture community and becoming a stellar healer and acupuncturist in your own right. Dawn Chitwood Rivers, you so reliably smooth out the kinks of our online presence and support our work while keeping your good cheer and humor intact. Peter Dechar, thanks for our shared delight in the wit, whimsy, and wisdom of Lao Tzu and for reminding us every so often to get the frog out of the well and out to the open sea.

Finally, to our home fire family—ally and familiar, Professor, our magical cat with the Taiji on her nose. She has kept us grounded when we lost our way and is a constant reminder of the abiding wisdom of the animal body. David Adler and Nina Wish Adler, who have brought the miracle of Diana Chava into our lives, you give us reason to keep on keeping on.

Medicinal Sources

Here is a list of the primary sources we use to obtain medicinals mentioned in this book. There are many others, and we'd be delighted if you share your own discoveries through our online community at *anewpossibility.com*.

Flower Essences

Flower Essence Services
P.O. Box 1769
Nevada City, CA 95959
800-548-0075
info@flowersociety.org
www.fesflowers.com

Healing Herbs, Ltd.
Walterstone
Hereford HR2 0DX
United Kingdom
+44 (0) 1873.890218
info@healingherbs.co.uk
www.healingherbs.co.uk

Oceans and Rivers—Essentials flower essence blends
718-913-0037
Lindsay@OceansandRivers.com
www.OceansandRivers.com

Nelson Bach USA, Ltd.
21 High Street, Suite 302
North Andover, MA 01845
800-319-9151
USACustomerService@nelsons.net
www.nelsons.net

Tree Frog Farm (offer essences with nonalcoholic red shiso leaf base)
3679 Sunrise Road
Lummi Island, WA 98262
(360) 758-7260
info@treefrogfarm.com
www.treefrogfarm.com

Wonderworks
25 Baldwin Street
Toronto, ON M5T 1L1
Canada
416-323-3131
800-329-0757 (International)
www.gowonderworks.com

Essential Oils

Essential Therapeutics
39 Melverton Drive
Hallam, VICTORIA 3803
Australia
03 8795 7720
www.essentialtherapeutics.com.au

Floracopeia
13100 Grass Valley Avenue,
Suite D
Grass Valley, CA 95945
866-417-1149
support@floracopeia.com
www.floracopeia.com

Original Swiss Aromatics
P.O. Box 6842
San Rafael, CA 94903
415-479-9120
www.originalswissaromatics.com

Reader's Guide Available

We believe that healing is a group activity. The power to transform or discover the broader meaning of an illness or suffering increases exponentially when people gather together to share their experiences and support each other's commitment to growth and change.

One effective way to take your Inner Work deeper is to download our Reader's Guide to *The Alchemy of Inner Work* and gather regularly, either in-person or virtually, with one or more people who are also reading the book. Turn your group into an alchemical laboratory! Read a chapter, discuss the questions, explore the practices on your own, and then gather again to talk about your personal experiences and learning.

As we emphasize throughout the book, alchemy is not a quick fix. It is an unfolding process that takes dedication and self-love, an art and a craft of the soul that happens in and through relationship over time. The rewards of this effort, while often unpredictable and surprising to the rational mind, are of value beyond measure and can help you transform the chaos and challenges of life into the gold of new possibilities.

You will find the Reader's Guide here as a free download: *https://bit.ly/Readers-Guide* or, if you would like to benefit from engagement with the Reader's Guide within a facilitate virtual group context, join our dedicated community at *www.anewpossibility.com*.

Bibliography

Blome, Gotz. *Advanced Bach Flower Therapy.* VT: Healing Arts Press, 1999.

Brown, Adrienne Maree. *Emergent Strategy: Shaping Change, Changing Worlds.* Chico, CA.: AK Press, 2017.

Cheak, Aaron, ed. *Alchemical Traditions: From Antiquity to Avant-Garde.* Melbourne, Australia: Numen Books, 2013.

Christie, Anthony. *Chinese Mythology.* Middlesex, England: Hamlyn Publishing Group Limited, 1968.

Cleary, Thomas, trans. *The Secret of the Golden Flower.* San Francisco: HarperSanFrancisco, 1991.

Cornell, Ann Weiser. *The Power of Focusing: A Practical Guide to Emotional Self-Healing.* Oakland, CA: New Harbinger Publications, 1996.

Craydon, Deborah, and Warren Bellows. *Floral Acupuncture: Applying the Flower Essences of Dr. Bach to Acupuncture Sites.* Berkeley, CA: The Crossing Press, 2005.

Dechar, Lorie Eve. *Five Spirits: Alchemical Acupuncture for Psychological and Spiritual Healing.* New York: Chiron/Lantern Books, 2006.

Eisenstein, Charles. *Climate: A New Story.* Berkeley, CA: North Atlantic Books, 2018.

———. *The More Beautiful World Our Hearts Know is Possible.* Berkeley, CA: North Atlantic Books, 2013.

Evola, Julius. *The Hermetic Tradition.* Rochester, VT: Inner Traditions International, 1995.

Fabricius, Johannes. *Alchemy: The Medieval Alchemists and their Royal Art.* London: Diamond Books, 1994.

Gebser, Jean. *The Ever-Present Origin.* Athens, OH: Ohio University Press, 1985.

Govinda, Lama Anagarika. *The Inner Structure of the I Ching: The Book of Transformations.* San Francisco: Wheelwright Press, 1981.

Haddon, Genia Pauli. *Uniting Sex Self & Spirit.* Scotland, CT: PLUS Publications, 1993.

Hauck, Dennis William. *The Emerald Tablet: Alchemy for Personal Transformation.* New York: Penguin Arkana, 1999.

———. *Working with the Metals.* Retrieved from *https://azothalchemy.org/ metals.htm*

Hillman, James. *A Blue Fire.* New York: Harper & Row, 1991.

HO, Mae-Wan. *The Rainbow and the Worm: The Physics of Organisms.* Singapore: World Scientific, 2008.

Jensen, Derrick. *A Language Older Than Words.* White River Junction, VT: Chelsea Green Publishing Company, 2004.

Johnson, Robert A. *Inner Work: Using Dreams & Active Imagination for Personal Growth.* San Francisco: HarperSanFrancisco, 1986.

Jung, C. G. *Alchemical Studies.* Princeton, NJ: Bollingen Press, 1967.

———. *Archetypes of the Collective Unconscious.* Princeton, NJ: Bollingen Press, 1959.

———. *Psychology and Alchemy.* Princeton, NJ: Princeton University Press, 1968.

Kingsley, Peter. *Catafalque: Carl Jung and The End of Humanity.* London: Catafalque Press, 2018.

Klocek, Dennis. *The Seer's Handbook: A Guide to Higher Perception.* Great Barrington, MA: Steiner Books, 2005.

Klossowski de Rola, Stanislas. *Alchemy: The Secret Art.* London: Thames and Hudson, 1997.

Kohn, Livia, ed. *Taoism Handbook.* Netherlands: Die Deutsche Bibliothek/Brill Academic Publishers, 2000.

———, ed. *Living Authentically: Daoist Contributions to Modern Psychology.* Dunedin, FL: Three Pines Press, 2011.

Larre, Claude. *The Way of Heaven: Neijing suwen.* Cambridge, UK: Monkey Press, 1994.

Larre, Claude, and Elizabeth Rochat de la Vallée. *The Heart: The Lingshu*. Cambridge, UK Monkey Press, 1996.

———. *Huang Di Nei Jing Su Wen: The Secret Treatise of the Spiritual Orchid*. Unrevised transcript of seminar presented at Ricci Institute, published by British Register of Oriental Medicine, 1985.

———. *The Lung*. London: Monkey Press, 2001.

———. *Rooted in Spirit: The Heart of Chinese Medicine*. Translated from French by Sarah Stang. New York: Station Hill Press, 1995.

Loewe, Michael. *Chinese Ideas of Life and Death: Faith, Myth and Reason in the Han Period (202 BC - Ad 220)*. London: George Allen & Unwin Ltd., 1982.

Macfarlane, Robert. *Underland: A Deep Time Journey*. New York: W. W. Norton & Company, 2019.

Mead, G.R.S. *The Doctrine of the Subtle Body*. Whitefish, MT: Kessinger Publishing Company, 2007.

Mehung, John A. *A Demonstration of Nature: Made to the Erring Alchemists, and Complaining of the Sophists and Other False Teachers*. Calgary: Theophania Publishing, 2011.

Mojay, Gabriel. *A\omatherapy for Healing the Spirit*. Rochester, VT: Healing Arts Press, 1997.

Needham, Joseph. "The Cosmology of Early China." *Ancient Cosmologies*. Cameron Blacker and Michael Loewe, eds. London: George Allen & Unwin Ltd., 1975.

Onians, R. B. *The Origins of European Thought About the Body, the Mind, the Soul, the World, Time, and Fate*. Cambridge, MA: Cambridge University Press, 1998.

Powers, Richard. *The Overstory*. New York: W. W. Norton & Company, Inc., 2018.

Prum, Richard. *The Evolution of Beauty: How Darwin's Forgotten Theory of Mate Choice Shapes the Animal World-and Us*. New York: Doubleday, 2017.

Ramsay, Jay. *Alchemy: The Art of Transformation*. London: Thorsons, 1997.

Ritsema, Rudolf and Stephen Karcher, trans. *I Ching*. Dorset, England: Element Books, 1994.

Robinet, Isabelle. *Taoism: The Growth of a Religion*. Stanford, CT: Stanford University Press, 1997.

Rochat de la Vallee, Elisabeth. *Wu Xing: The Five Elements in Classical Chinese Texts*. Cambridge, UK: Monkey Press, 2009.

Ronnberg, Ami, ed. *The Book of Symbols: Reflections on Archetypal Images*. Cologne, Germany: Taschen Press, 2010.

Roszak, Theodore, Mary Gomes, and Allen Kanner, eds. *Ecopsychology: Restoring the Earth Healing the Mind*. San Francisco: Sierra Club Books, 1995.

Rudhyar, Dane. *Person Centered Astrology*. Santa Fe, NM: Aurora Press, 1980.

Scheffer, Mechthild. *Bach Flower Therapy: Theory and Practice*. Rochester, VT: Healing Arts Press, 1984.

Schwartz-Salant, Nathan, ed. *Jung on Alchemy*. London: Routledge Press, 1995.

———. *The Mystery of Human Relationship*. London/New York: Routledge, 1998.

———. *The Order-Disorder Paradox*. Berkeley, CA: North Atlantic Books, 2017.

Sowton, Christopher. *The Dreamworking Manual: A Guide to Using Dreams in Health Care*. Toronto: Christopher Sowton, 2013.

Star, Jonathan, trans. Lao Tzu. *Tao Te Ching: The Definitive Edition*. New York: Jeremy P. Tarcher/Putnam, 2001.

Travers, P. L. *What the Bee Knows: Reflections on Myth, Symbol and Story*. New York: Arkana Penguin Book, 1993.

Unschuld, Paul. *Medicine in China: A History of Ideas*. Berkeley, CA: University of California Press, 1985.

van der Kolk, Bessel. *The Body Keeps the Score: Brain, Mind, and Body in the Healing of Trauma*. New York: Penguin Books, 2014.

Veith, Ilza, trans. *The Yellow Emperor's Classic of Internal Medicine*. Berkeley, CA: University of California Press, 1972.

von Franz, Marie Louise. *Alchemical Active Imagination*. Boston: Shambhala, 1997.

Waite, Edward, ed. *The Hermetic Museum: Twenty-Two Most Celebrated Chemical Tracts*. York, ME: Samuel Weiser, 1999.

The Alchemy of Inner Work

Watson, Burton, trans. *Chuang Tzu: Basic Writings.* New York: Columbia University Press, 1996.

Wenlin Institute. *Wenlin Software for Learning Chinese* (including ABC Dictionary by John DeFrancis). Version 2.0: *www.wenlin.com*, 1998.

Wilhelm, Richard, trans. *T'ai I Chin Hua Tsung Chih / The Secret of the Golden Flower.* Rendered into English by Cary Baynes. London: Kegan Paul, Trench, Trubner & Co. Ltd., 1942.

Wilhelm, Richard, trans. *The I Ching.* Rendered into English by Cary Baynes. Princeton, NJ: Bollingen Series, Princeton University Press, 1950.

Watts, Alan. *Tao: The Watercourse Way.* New York: Pantheon Books, 1975.

Wolkstein, Diane and Samuel Kramer, trans. *Inanna: Queen of Heaven and Earth.* New York: Harper and Row, 1983.

Worsley, J. R. *Acupuncture: Is It for You?* Great Britain: Element Books, 1973.

————. *Classical Five-Element Acupuncture: The Five Elements and Officials.* United Kingdom: J. R. and J. B. Worsley, 1998.

Wu, John C. H., trans. Lao Tzu. *Tao Teh Ching.* Edited by Paul K. T. Sih. New York: St. John's University Press, 1961.

Ying-Shih Yu. "O Soul, Come Back!" A Study in the Changing Conceptions of the Soul and Afterlife in Pre-Buddhist China. Harvard Journal of Asiatic Studies. Vol. 7. Cambridge, MA: Harvard-Yenching Institute, 1987.

To Our Readers

Weiser Books, an imprint of Red Wheel/Weiser, publishes books across the entire spectrum of occult, esoteric, speculative, and New Age subjects. Our mission is to publish quality books that will make a difference in people's lives without advocating any one particular path or field of study. We value the integrity, originality, and depth of knowledge of our authors.

Our readers are our most important resource, and we appreciate your input, suggestions, and ideas about what you would like to see published.

Visit our website at *www.redwheelweiser.com* to learn about our upcoming books and free downloads, and be sure to go to *www.redwheelweiser.com/newsletter* to sign up for newsletters and exclusive offers.

You can also contact us at *info@rwwbooks.com* or at
Red Wheel/Weiser, LLC
65 Parker Street, Suite 7
Newburyport, MA 01950